PARAMEDIC PORTFOLIO WORKBOOK

AF882448

TABLE OF CONTENTS

Introduction

Part 1 - Scenarios:

Part 2 - Scenario and Skills Tracking:

Introduction

Preparing to be a paramedic is an arduous but rewarding journey. As you progress on this journey you will develop both psychomotor skills and as importantly critical thinking and reasoning abilities to reinforce the skills. The process of completing the Paramedic Portfolio is likewise a very involved task. The goal of this T3 Paramedic Portfolio workbook is twofold: to serve as an aid in the development of your portfolio but also to help develop the lifelong skill of deliberate practice. Deliberate practice is the ability to analyze your actions upon reflection and adjust as necessary as you learn through trial and error. The T3 System is a set of tools that provide a robust scenario framework for both instructor led and peer scenarios. Scenarios are an incredible tool to supplement field experience. Adults learn by doing and "Train as we Treat" is a proven learning methodology .

Workbook Organization

The heart of this manual is centered on scenario performance and the book contains 21 chapters developed around particular scenario topics. Each chapter contains an overview of the case, pathophysiology related to the condition, skills checklists , debriefing and critical thinking questions and PCR's to capture performance data. Documentation is a foundational skill in EMS and the workbook serves as a tool to capture and track performance for later input.

The CAAHEP 2019 Minimum Student Competencies define the number and type of learning experiences students must complete on their Paramedic learning journey. The T3 System and this workbook were developed to track these skills in a convenient format. In the 2nd section of the workbook you will find handy tracking grids that will guide you through the process of completing the necessary learning steps.

Online Resources

We believe that peer scenarios can play a strong role in your development. As a companion to the T3 System we have developed a Team Scenario Facilitator (TSF) elearning credential. By understanding core scenario performance, development and debriefing you will be more able to benefit from these intensive learning experiences. Learn more about the TSF credential at www.t3sim.com

PART 1-

SCENARIOS

ADULT CARDIAC RHYTHM DISTURBANCE

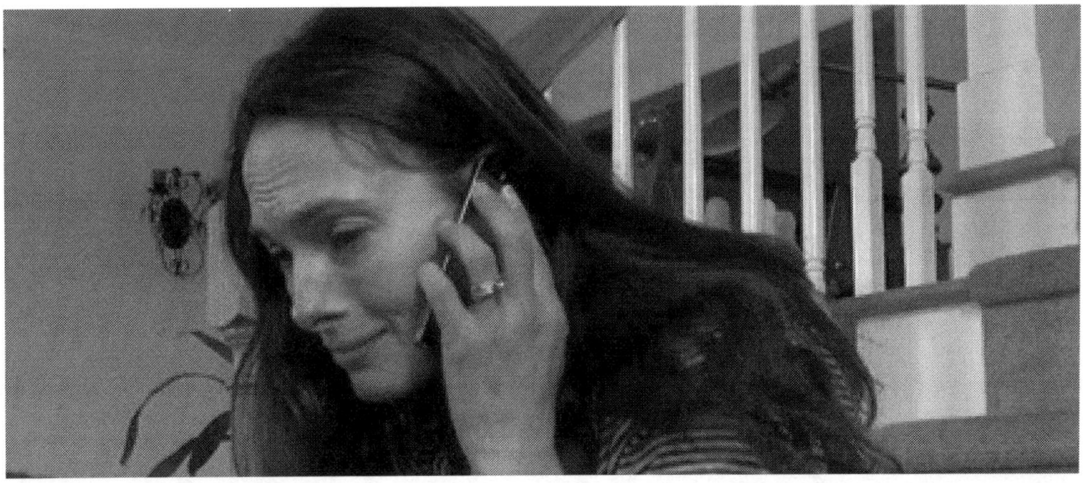

44 Y/O FEMALE, COMPLAINING OF RACING HEARTBEAT

DISPATCH
Location: Suburban home
Type of situation:Rapid heart rate
Number of patients: 1
Hazards: No hazards

OBJECTIVES

a. Assessment of the patient, assessment of the scene.
b. Understanding of the multiple causes rapid heart rates.
c. Understanding of the multiple arrhythmias above a rate of 150.
d. Prioritization of interventions.
e. Recognition of signs and symptoms of an unstable arrhythmia.
f. Performance of appropriate interventions.
g. Demonstrate effective teamwork.

SCENE SIZE-UP	
OVERALL SAFETY	SCENE IS SAFE
MOI / NOI	RAPID HEART RATE
RESOURCES	ALS RESPONSE
C-SPINE	NO SIGNS OF TRAUMA

PATHOPHYSIOLOGY

Overview:

Heart rates above 150 may be a result of many causes. It is dependent upon the provider determining if the rate is the result of the cause, or the cause is the rate. This will determine the treatment. Sinus tachycardia of 150 is at the upper limit and can be a function of an underlying cause. These causes can be hypovolemia, sepsis, infection, excessive metabolic response, pain, or hypercarbia. Treatment is treating the underlying cause of the tachycardia.

A rate of 150 bpm can be from a primary cardiac cause. SVT, Atrial tachycardia, ventricular tachycardia and aberrantly conducted SVT can all present at 150 bpm. The first determination must be if the patient is stable with this rate. If the patient is unstable with ongoing chest pain, signs of hypoperfusion, decreased LOC, then the patient must be immediately cardioverted.

If the patient is stable with one of these arrhythmias then the type of arrhythmia will determine the treatment. If the patient with the arrhythmia is stable then pharmacological treatment is indicated. Adenosine is indicated for SVT, Diltiazem is indicted for most A-Fib and A-Flutter, and

Amiodarone is indicated for V-Tach.

Tachycardia: Performance

Performance Checklist Role:

Start Time: End Time:

Expected Actions	Time	2	1	0	N/A
1. Scene Size-up*					
2. PS: ABCs					
3. PS: 02 NRB					
4. PS: Aspirin					
5. SA: Vitals					
6. SA: Blood sugar					
7. SA: Obtain EKG*					
8. Differential DX- SVT*					
9. TI: Vagal maneuvres					
10. TI: IV access*					
11. TI: 6 mg Adenosine*					
12. Reassessment					
13. TI: Diltiazem*					
14. Transport*					
AMBULANCE					
15. Reassessment					
16. Report					
TEAMWORK/LEADERSHIP					
1. Coordination of Treatment					
2. Communication					
3. Situational Awareness					
4. Affect					
5. Overall					

*actions are mandatory

SELF EVALUATION: ☐ Successful ☐ Unsuccessful

SCORE: /42

NOTES:

Potentially Harmful/Dangerous actions (omission, commission, sequencing):

C DEBRIEFING

Debriefing Questions:

1. How did feel throughout the simulation experience?
2. What were your primary diagnoses in this scenario?
3. Did you feel you had the knowledge and skills to care for this patient? Why/ why not?
4. What were your priority assessments and interventions?
5. What outcomes did you measure?
6. What did you do well?
7. What was missed? What would you have done differently?
8. Is there anything else you would like to discuss?

Critical Thinking:

1. What was the original arrhythmia?

2. Should this patient have been cardioverted?

3. When should A-Fib be treated?

T3 SIMULATION SYSTEM

Tachycardia: Performance

Performance Checklist Role:

Start Time: End Time:

Expected Actions	Time	2	1	0	N/A
1. Scene Size-up*					
2. PS: ABCs					
3. PS: 02 NRB					
4. PS: Aspirin					
5. SA: Vitals					
6. SA: Blood sugar					
7. SA: Obtain EKG*					
8. Differential DX- SVT unstable*					
9. TI: Vagal maneuvres					
10. TI: IV access*					
11. TI: Cardioversion *					
12. Reassessment					
13. TI: *					
14. Transport* AMBULANCE					
15. Reassessment					
16. Report					
TEAMWORK/LEADERSHIP					
1. Coordination of Treatment					
2. Communication					
3. Situational Awareness					
4. Affect*					
5. Overall					

*actions are mandatory

SELF EVALUATION: ☐ Successful ☐ Unsuccessful

SCORE: /42

NOTES:

Potentially Harmful/Dangerous actions (omission, commission, sequencing):

C DEBRIEFING

Debriefing Questions:

1. How did feel throughout the simulation experience?
2. What were your primary diagnoses in this scenario?
3. Did you feel you had the knowledge and skills to care for this patient? Why/ why not?
4. What were your priority assessments and interventions?
5. What outcomes did you measure?
6. What did you do well?
7. What was missed? What would you have done differently?
8. Is there anything else you would like to discuss?

Critical Thinking:

1. What was the original arrhythmia?
2. Should this patient have been cardioverted?
3. When should A-Fib be treated?

EMS PATIENT CARE REPORT (PCR) Scenario:

PATIENT INFORMATION

Name:
Age:
Sex:
Weight: Kg (lb)

Allergies:
Medications:
Past Medical History:
Chief Complaint:

VITAL SIGNS

Time:	BP:	Pulse:	Respiration:	Sao_2:
Time:	BP:	Pulse:	Respiration:	Sao_2:
Time:	BP:	Pulse:	Respiration:	Sao_2:

PHYSICAL / NEUROLOGICAL EXAM

LOC:
Oriented:
GCS:
Pupils:
Sensory/Motor:
Facial Droop:
Speech:

Skin:
HEENT:
Neck:
Chest:
Respiratory:
Cardiovascular:
EKG:

AB/GI:
Pelvis:
GU:
Posterior :
Extremities:
Psychiatric:
GLU:

CHIEF COMPLAINT

HISTORY OF PRESENT ILLNESS

NOTES

EMS PATIENT CARE REPORT (PCR) Scenario:

PATIENT INFORMATION

Name:	Allergies:
Age:	Medications:
Sex:	Past Medical History:
Weight: Kg (lb)	Chief Complaint:

VITAL SIGNS

Time:	BP:	Pulse:	Respiration:	Sao_2:
Time:	BP:	Pulse:	Respiration:	Sao_2:
Time:	BP:	Pulse:	Respiration:	Sao_2:

PHYSICAL / NEUROLOGICAL EXAM

LOC:	Skin:	AB/GI:
Oriented:	HEENT:	Pelvis:
GCS:	Neck:	GU:
Pupils:	Chest:	Posterior :
Sensory/Motor:	Respiratory:	Extremities:
Facial Droop:	Cardiovascular:	Psychiatric:
Speech:	EKG:	GLU:

CHIEF COMPLAINT

HISTORY OF PRESENT ILLNESS

NOTES

ADULT DIABETIC EMERGENCY

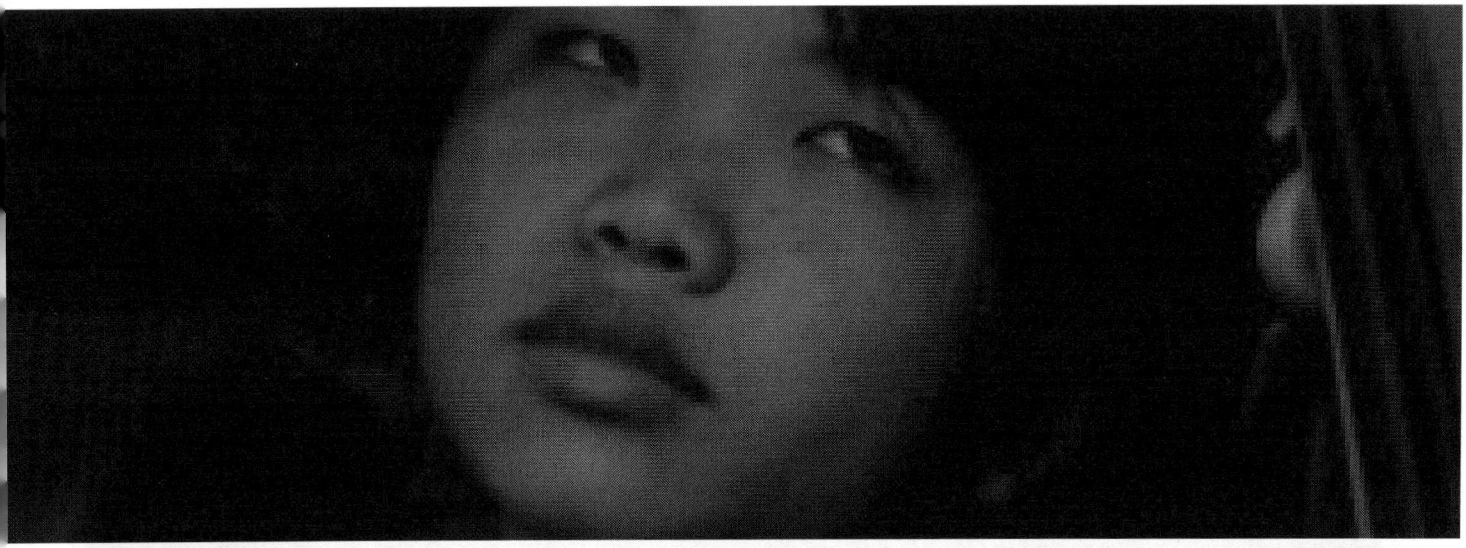

21 Y/O MALE, ALTERED MENTAL STATUS

DISPATCH
Location: Parking lot
Type of situation:AMS
Number of patients: 1
Hazards: No hazards

OBJECTIVES
1. Assessment of the patient
2. Prioritize interventions
3. Recognition of hypoglycemia
4. reat symptomatic hypoglycemia
5. Assess effectiveness of interventions
6 Recognize need for priority transport
7. Demonstrate high performance teamwork

SCENE SIZE-UP	
OVERALL SAFETY	SCENE IS SAFE
MOI / NOI	ALTERED MENTAL STATUS, POSSIBLE STROKE
RESOURCES	ALS RESPONSE
C-SPINE	NO SIGNS OF TRAUMA

PATHOPHYSIOLOGY

Overview:

Hypoglycemia onset is rapid and deteriorates rapidly. A patient that cannot swallow on command cannot protect his/her airway and should not be given oral glucose. Responding to voice is an altered level of consciousness. The brain cannot store energy and relies on the glucose in the blood for a constant supply. At the point where the glucose in the blood drops below a normal level, several symptoms may occur. Altered consciousness, seizures, one sided paralysis, unconsciousness. Cardiac abnormalities can also occur. A blood sugar level below 10 may cause death. Unconscious diabetics also do not produce heat and pass through a diaphoretic stage. If left untreated they are cold and wet and become hypothermic. This slows the absorption of the glucose administered and also makes IV access difficult. Once they become aroused there will be a period of shivering once they reach a core temperature of 92 degrees. During prolonged low blood sugar events, the pancreas releases glucagon which travels to the liver, interacting to release more circulating glucose. If the liver stores are depleated, glucagon will not help. There is evidence that very low blood sugar for a prolonged period may cause a late release of the remaining liver stores creating a spike in LOC for a brief time. This is believed to be a protective mechanism.

Hyperglycemia has a slow onset and usually presents with frequent urination, dehydration, warm skin, furrowed tongue (brown and fuzzy). Sweet breath smell from keytones (breaking down of fat metabolism). History of recent illness.

T3 SIMULATION SYSTEM

Diabetic: Performance

Performance Checklist Role:

Start Time: End Time:

Expected Actions	Time	2	1	0	N/A
1. Scene size-up					
2. Primary Survey: LOC, CC, HPI					
3. Primary Survey: ABCs					
4. TI: 100% 02 NRB 15 lpm					
5. SA: Blood Glucose 46					
6. Secondary Assessment: Vitals					
7. Differential DX: Hypoglycemia					
8. TI: IV access					
9. TI: Dextrose 25 grams sugar					
10. Reassessment					
11. Transport: Non-emergent					
12. Reassessment : BS 100					
13. Keep patient warm					
14. Affect: Hospital requirement					
15. Report					
TEAMWORK/LEADERSHIP					
1. Coordination of Treatment					
2. Communication					
3. Situational Awareness					
4. Affect					
5. Overall					

SELF EVALUATION: ☐ Successful ☐ Unsuccessful

SCORE: /40

NOTES:

C DEBRIEFING

Debriefing Questions:

1. What happened?
2. How did you feel throughout the simulation experience?
3. What were your priority assessments and interventions?
4. What did you do well?
5. What was missed? What would you have done differently?
6. What additional information would you need?
7. Is there anything else you would like to discuss?

Critical Thinking

1. Why did this patient not get oral glucose?
2. What if IV cannot be established?
3. Could this person not have been transported?

T3 SIMULATION SYSTEM

Diabetic: Performance

Performance Checklist Role:

Start Time:	End Time:

Expected Actions	Time	2	1	0	N/A
1. Scene size-up					
2. Primary Survey: LOC, CC, HPI					
3. Primary Survey: ABCs					
4. TI: 100% 02 NRB 15 lpm					
5. SA: Blood Glucose					
6. Secondary Assessment:					
Vitals					
7. Differential DX:DKA					
8. TI: IV access					
9. TI: Normal Saline					
10. Reassessment					
11. Transport: Non-emergent					
12. Reassessment :					
13. Report					
TEAMWORK/LEADERSHIP					
1. Coordination of Treatment					
2. Communication					
3. Situational Awareness					
4. Affect					
5. Overall					

SELF EVALUATION: ☐ Successful ☐ Unsuccessful

SCORE: /36

NOTES:

C DEBRIEFING

Debriefing Questions:

1. What happened?
2. How did you feel throughout the simulation experience?
3. What were your priority assessments and interventions?
4. What did you do well?
5. What was missed? What would you have done differently?
6. What additional information would you need?
7. Is there anything else you would like to discuss?

Critical Thinking

1. What is the mechanism of dehydration in DKA patients?
2. What are the main components of prehospital DKA management?

EMS PATIENT CARE REPORT (PCR) Scenario:

PATIENT INFORMATION

Name:	Allergies:
Age:	Medications:
Sex:	Past Medical History:
Weight: Kg (lb)	Chief Complaint:

VITAL SIGNS

Time:	BP:	Pulse:	Respiration:	Sao_2:
Time:	BP:	Pulse:	Respiration:	Sao_2:
Time:	BP:	Pulse:	Respiration:	Sao_2:

PHYSICAL / NEUROLOGICAL EXAM

LOC:	Skin:	AB/GI:
Oriented:	HEENT:	Pelvis:
GCS:	Neck:	GU:
Pupils:	Chest:	Posterior :
Sensory/Motor:	Respiratory:	Extremities:
Facial Droop:	Cardiovascular:	Psychiatric:
Speech:	EKG:	GLU:

CHIEF COMPLAINT

HISTORY OF PRESENT ILLNESS

NOTES

EMS PATIENT CARE REPORT (PCR) Scenario:

PATIENT INFORMATION

Name:	Allergies:
Age:	Medications:
Sex:	Past Medical History:
Weight: Kg (lb)	Chief Complaint:

VITAL SIGNS

Time:	BP:	Pulse:	Respiration:	Sao_2:
Time:	BP:	Pulse:	Respiration:	Sao_2:
Time:	BP:	Pulse:	Respiration:	Sao_2:

PHYSICAL / NEUROLOGICAL EXAM

LOC:	Skin:	AB/GI:
Oriented:	HEENT:	Pelvis:
GCS:	Neck:	GU:
Pupils:	Chest:	Posterior :
Sensory/Motor:	Respiratory:	Extremities:
Facial Droop:	Cardiovascular:	Psychiatric:
Speech:	EKG:	GLU:

CHIEF COMPLAINT

HISTORY OF PRESENT ILLNESS

NOTES

ADULT OVERDOSE

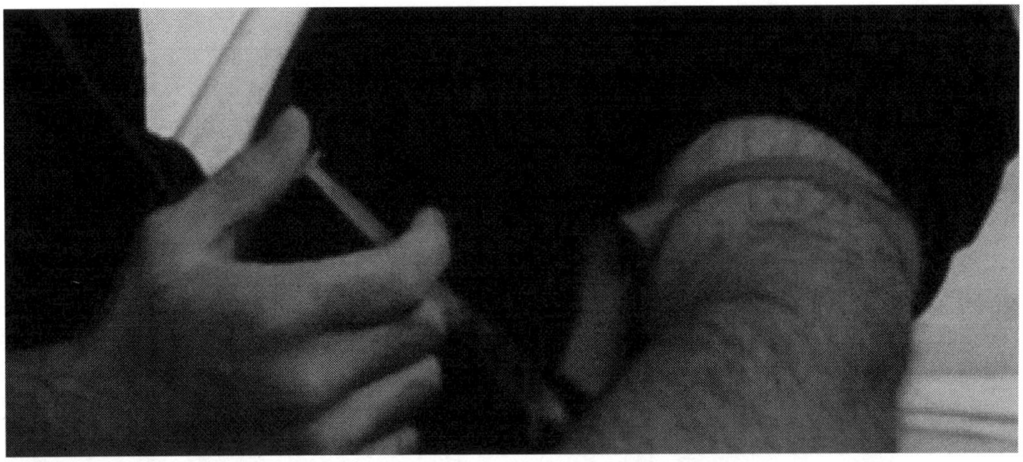

UNRESPONSIVE 25 Y/O MALE POSSIBLE OVERDOSE

DISPATCH

Location: Low rent motel room.
Type of situation: Unconscious
Number of patients: 1
Hazards: A syringe and open needle next to patient

OBJECTIVES

1. Discuss Scene Safety considerations for a possible overdose patient
2. Describe the Assessment and Treatment of a patient with a possible overdose
3. Understand the role of Airway Management in the possible overdose patient
4. Prioritize and perform appropriate interventions.
5. Describe the steps in the administration of intranasal medications
6. Demonstrate effective teamwork.

SCENE SIZE-UP	
OVERALL SAFETY	POLICE ARE ON SCENE
MOI / NOI	NARCOTIC OVERDOSE
RESOURCES	ALS RESPONSE
C-SPINE	NO SIGNS OF TRAUMA

PATHOPHYSIOLOGY

Overview:

While several different types of drugs can be administered IV, narcotics are one of the few that causes respiratory depression, a decreased level of consciousness and pinpoint pupils. It is not important to identify which type of narcotic was used, as the treatment is the same. The triad of pinpoint pupils, respiratory depression, and decreased level of consciousness should immediately lead the responder to managing the airway and providing respiratory support. Even if respiratory effort is present, it is frequently too shallow to maintain oxygenation. BVM is critical. Often a nasal trumpet works very well in keeping the airway open. Narcan should be given slowly, and titrated to respiratory effort and SaO2.

Scene safety should be paramount. A supportive non-judgmental approach is ideal.

OD- Scenario Checklist 1

T3 SIMULATION SYSTEM

Performance Checklist Role: | Start Time: End Time:

Expected Actions	Time	2	1	0	N/A
1. Scene size-up *					
2. PS: ABCs					
3. TI : BVM Airway Management*					
4. SA: Vitals					
5. SA: Blood Sugar					
6. Differential DX: Opioid Overdose*					
7. TI: Narcan IN*					
8. Reassessment incl monitor					
9. Transport					
10. Reassessment*					
11. IV Access *					
12. IV NARCAN*					
13. Reassessment					
14. Report					
TEAMWORK/LEADERSHIP					
1. Coordination of Treatment					
2. Communication					
3. Situational Awareness					
4. Affect					
5. Overall					

SELF EVALUATION: ☐ Successful ☐ Unsuccessful

SCORE: /38

NOTES: including Critical Items

REFLECTION

Debriefing Questions:

1. How did you feel throughout the simulation experience?

2. What were your primary diagnoses in this scenario?

3. Did you feel you had the knowledge and skills to care for this patient? Why/ why not?

4. What were your priority assessments and interventions?

5. What did you do well?

7. What was missed? What would you have done differently?

Critical Thinking

1. What is the safest way to give Narcan?

2. Why do you titrate the dose of Narcan to the respiratory status and not the LOC?

OD- Scenario Checklist 2

Performance Checklist | **Role:** | **Start Time:** | **End Time:**

Expected Actions	Time	2	1	0	N/A
1. Scene size-up *					
2. PS: ABCs					
3. TI : BVM Airway Management*					
4. SA: Vitals					
5. SA: Blood Sugar/ Monitor					
6. Differential DX: TCA Overdose*					
7. TI: IV Access and Fluids					
8. Reassessment incl monitor					
9. TI: Sodium Bicarb *					
10. Transport					
11. Reassessment*					
12. Report					
TEAMWORK/LEADERSHIP					
1. Coordination of Treatment					
2. Communication					
3. Situational Awareness					
4. Affect					
5. Overall					

SELF EVALUATION: ☐ Successful ☐ Unsuccessful

SCORE: /34

NOTES: including Critical Items

REFLECTION

Debriefing Questions:

1. How did you feel throughout the simulation experience?

2. What were your primary diagnoses in this scenario?

3. Did you feel you had the knowledge and skills to care for this patient? Why/ why not?

4. What were your priority assessments and interventions?

5. What did you do well?

7. What was missed? What would you have done differently?

Critical Thinking

1. What does a widened QRS indicate?

2. Explain the effects of sodium bicarb.

EMS PATIENT CARE REPORT (PCR) Scenario:

PATIENT INFORMATION

Name: Age: Sex: Weight: Kg (lb)	Allergies: Medications: Past Medical History: Chief Complaint:

VITAL SIGNS

Time:	BP:	Pulse:	Respiration:	Sao_2:
Time:	BP:	Pulse:	Respiration:	Sao_2:
Time:	BP:	Pulse:	Respiration:	Sao_2:

PHYSICAL / NEUROLOGICAL EXAM

LOC: Oriented: GCS: Pupils: Sensory/Motor: Facial Droop: Speech:	Skin: HEENT: Neck: Chest: Respiratory: Cardiovascular: EKG:	AB/GI: Pelvis: GU: Posterior : Extremities: Psychiatric: GLU:

CHIEF COMPLAINT

HISTORY OF PRESENT ILLNESS

NOTES

EMS PATIENT CARE REPORT (PCR) Scenario:

PATIENT INFORMATION

Name:	Allergies:
Age:	Medications:
Sex:	Past Medical History:
Weight: Kg (lb)	Chief Complaint:

VITAL SIGNS

Time:	BP:	Pulse:	Respiration:	Sao_2:
Time:	BP:	Pulse:	Respiration:	Sao_2:
Time:	BP:	Pulse:	Respiration:	Sao_2:

PHYSICAL / NEUROLOGICAL EXAM

LOC:	Skin:	AB/GI:
Oriented:	HEENT:	Pelvis:
GCS:	Neck:	GU:
Pupils:	Chest:	Posterior :
Sensory/Motor:	Respiratory:	Extremities:
Facial Droop:	Cardiovascular:	Psychiatric:
Speech:	EKG:	GLU:

CHIEF COMPLAINT

HISTORY OF PRESENT ILLNESS

NOTES

ADULT PSYCHIATRIC CONDITION

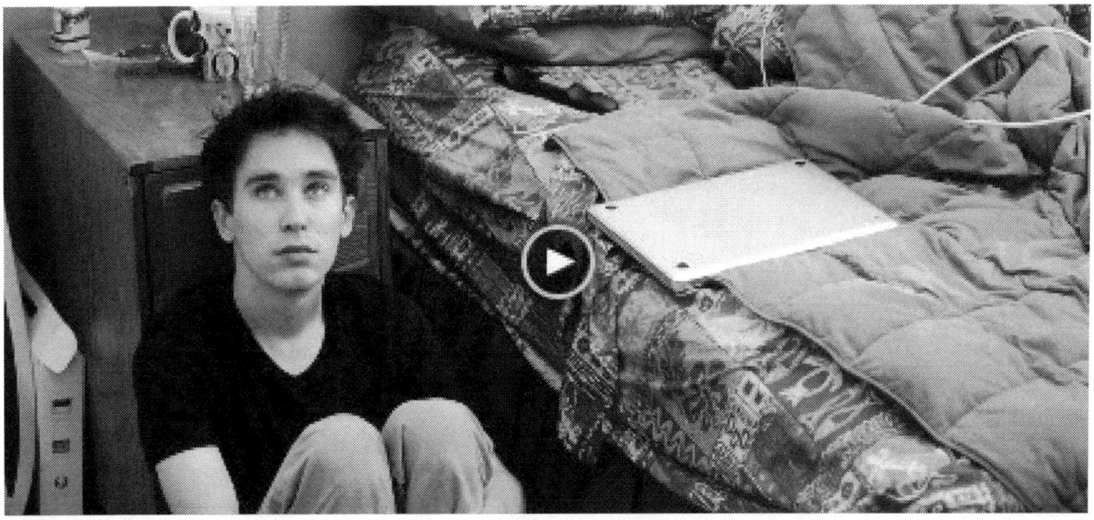

24 Y/O MALE, ALTERED MENTAL STATUS

DISPATCH
Location: Suburban home
Type of situation: AMS, possible psychiatric emergency
Number of patients: 1
Hazards: No hazards

OBJECTIVES
1. Scene safety
2. Understanding of the pathophysiology of Mental Illness
3. Prioritization and performance of appropriate interventions
4. Recognition the signs and symptoms of Mental Illness
5. Demonstration of compassion and non-judgmental attitude.
6. Demonstration of effective teamwork

SCENE SIZE-UP	
OVERALL SAFETY	SCENE IS SAFE, PD ON SCENE
MOI / NOI	ALTERED MENTAL STATUS, POSSIBLE PSYCHIATRIC EMERGENCY
RESOURCES	BLS RESPONSE
C-SPINE	NO SIGNS OF TRAUMA

PATHOPHYSIOLOGY

Overview:

Schizophrenia is a psychosis that usually presents in the 2nd decade of life. It is manifested by a loss of reality. The schizophrenic is unable to separate reality from distortions. Schizophrenia is a brain disorder that is thought to be partially genetic. It affects 1% of the population.This disorder is characterized by hallucinations- most commonly voices only heard by the patient, Delusions- beliefs that the patient may have that are not part of the culture. (Such as the TV is sending messages via commercials to the patient, or the government is reading their thoughts.) Thought Disorder- where higher level thinking is disorganized, not linear.

Some schizophrenics have delusions that people are out to hurt them, or that they should hurt other people. This is known as paranoid schizophrenia. This can be dangerous to responders.

Psychosis is treated with medications like Seroquel, Risperdal, and Haldol. Most patients are able to function while on medications, but frequently stop taking them. The responder should not participate in the delusion or hallucination; but since the delusion or hallucination are real to the patient they should not be dismissed either. Treatment is supportive, non-judgmental, and compassionate. Physical restraint should be planned out, executed swiftly, and confidently and is usually under the direction of the police.

Schizophrenia: Performance

Performance Checklist Role: | Start Time: End Time:

Expected Actions	Time	2	1	0	N/A
1. Scene SU: Address Safety *					
2. PS: CC, LOC, HPI					
3. PS: ABC					
4. SA: Vital Signs					
5. Blood Sugar					
6. Past Medical: History					
7. DD: Schizophrenia Exacerbation *					
8. Affect: Pt. Cooperation					
9. Transport: Non-emergent *					
10. Reassessment: ABCs, Vitals, Place Pt. on Monitor					
11. Restrain Patient *					
12. TI: Medication IM Versed *					
13. Reassessment					
14. Communication: Transparent Thinking					
15. Report					
TEAMWORK/LEADERSHIP					
1. Coordination					
2. Flexibility					
3. Communication					
4. Affect: Rapport & Support *					
5. Overall					

(*) actions are mandatory

SELF EVALUATION: ☐ Successful ☐ Unsuccessful | **SCORE:** /40

NOTES:

Potentially Harmful/ Dangerous Actions (omission, commission, sequencing):

C DEBRIEFING

Debriefing Questions:

1. How did you feel throughout the simulation experience?
2. What were your primary diagnoses in this scenario?
3. Did you feel you had the knowledge and skills to care for this patient? Why/ why not?
4. What were your priority assessments and interventions?
5. What outcomes did you measure?
6. What did you do well?
7. What was missed? What would you have done differently?
8. Is there anything else you would like to discuss?

Critical Thinking

1. How do you tell if the patient is going to be violent?

2. Are the hallucinations and delusions made up or real to the patient?

3. How do you think the best way is to handle a mentally ill patient?

Schizophrenia: Performance

Performance Checklist   Role: Start Time: End Time:

Expected Actions	Time	2	1	0	N/A
1. Scene SU: Address Safety *					
2. PS: CC, LOC, HPI					
3. PS: ABC					
4. SA: Vital Signs					
5. Blood Sugar					
6. Past Medical: History					
7. DD: Schizophrenia Exacerbation *					
8. Affect: Pt. Cooperation					
9. Transport: Non-emergent *					
10. Reassessment: ABCs, Vitals, Place Pt. on Monitor					
11. Restrain Patient *					
12. TI: Medication IM Versed *					
13. Reassessment					
14. Communication: Transparent Thinking					
!5. Report					
TEAMWORK/LEADERSHIP					
1. Coordination					
2. Flexibility					
3. Communication					
4. Affect: Rapport & Support *					
5. Overall					

(*) actions are mandatory

SELF EVALUATION: ☐ Successful ☐ Unsuccessful

SCORE: /40

NOTES:

Potentially Harmful/ Dangerous Actions (omission, commission, sequencing):

C DEBRIEFING

Debriefing Questions:

1. How did you feel throughout the simulation experience?
2. What were your primary diagnoses in this scenario?
3. Did you feel you had the knowledge and skills to care for this patient? Why/ why not?
4. What were your priority assessments and interventions?
5. What outcomes did you measure?
6. What did you do well?
7. What was missed? What would you have done differently?
8. Is there anything else you would like to discuss?

Critical Thinking

1. How do you tell if the patient is going to be violent?

2. Are the hallucinations and delusions made up or real to the patient?

3. How do you think the best way is to handle a mentally ill patient?

EMS PATIENT CARE REPORT (PCR) Scenario:

PATIENT INFORMATION

Name:	Allergies:
Age:	Medications:
Sex:	Past Medical History:
Weight: Kg (lb)	Chief Complaint:

VITAL SIGNS

Time:	BP:	Pulse:	Respiration:	Sao_2:
Time:	BP:	Pulse:	Respiration:	Sao_2:
Time:	BP:	Pulse:	Respiration:	Sao_2:

PHYSICAL / NEUROLOGICAL EXAM

LOC:	Skin:	AB/GI:
Oriented:	HEENT:	Pelvis:
GCS:	Neck:	GU:
Pupils:	Chest:	Posterior :
Sensory/Motor:	Respiratory:	Extremities:
Facial Droop:	Cardiovascular:	Psychiatric:
Speech:	EKG:	GLU:

CHIEF COMPLAINT

HISTORY OF PRESENT ILLNESS

NOTES

EMS PATIENT CARE REPORT (PCR) Scenario:

PATIENT INFORMATION

Name:	Allergies:
Age:	Medications:
Sex:	Past Medical History:
Weight: Kg (lb)	Chief Complaint:

VITAL SIGNS

Time:	BP:	Pulse:	Respiration:	Sao_2:
Time:	BP:	Pulse:	Respiration:	Sao_2:
Time:	BP:	Pulse:	Respiration:	Sao_2:

PHYSICAL / NEUROLOGICAL EXAM

LOC:	Skin:	AB/GI:
Oriented:	HEENT:	Pelvis:
GCS:	Neck:	GU:
Pupils:	Chest:	Posterior :
Sensory/Motor:	Respiratory:	Extremities:
Facial Droop:	Cardiovascular:	Psychiatric:
Speech:	EKG:	GLU:

CHIEF COMPLAINT

HISTORY OF PRESENT ILLNESS

NOTES

ADULT SEIZURE

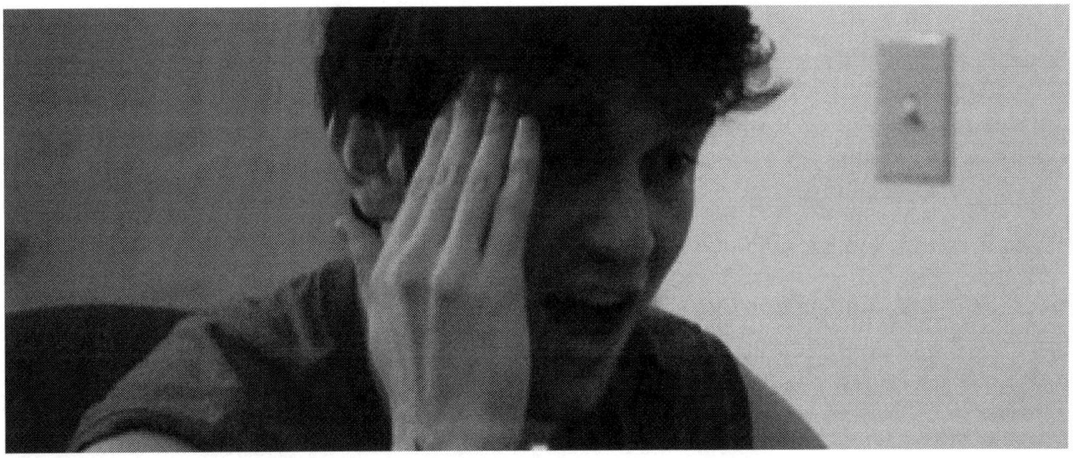

22 Y/O MALE, ACTIVE SEIZURE

DISPATCH
Location: Suburban apartment
Type of situation: Active seizure
Number of patients: 1
Hazards: No hazards

OBJECTIVES

a. Recognizing seizure and the need for a very calm setting.
b. Understanding of the pathophysiology of seizures.
c. Assessment of the seizing patient.
d. Prioritization and performance of appropriate interventions.
e. Performance of appropriate interventions.
f. Demonstration of effective teamwork.

SCENE SIZE-UP	
OVERALL SAFETY	SCENE IS SAFE
MOI / NOI	ACTIVE SEIZURE
RESOURCES	ALS RESPONSE
C-SPINE	UNKNOWN

PATHOPHYSIOLOGY

Overview:

Seizures (epilepsy) are a common disorder. A simple seizure is rarely a medical emergency. Seizures are classified by the activity of the seizure;

The most common are generalized seizures that involve motor activity of all the limbs. During a generalized seizure the patient is unconscious, and nonresponsive. Apnea is common during this type of seizure.

Partial/complex seizures present as motor activity (twitching) of a single limb/digit, single side of the body or of the face. During a partial/complex seizure the patient may be unconscious or unresponsive but awake.

Most seizures are self-limiting and are frequently over by the time EMS arrives. If the seizure activity is continuous or with little recovery time between seizures the patient is in status seizures.

Status seizures are a medical emergency, with airway and breathing as the major concern. Confirmation of adequate respiratory effort and pulse are critical during status seizures. Hypoxemia and dysrhythmias may result if the airway and breathing are not controlled.

The continuous muscle activity associated with status seizures can create lactic acidosis which causes additional respiratory compromise; products of muscle breakdown can damage the kidneys.

Almost any disorder can cause a seizure. It is critical to access the ABC's during and after the seizure to ensure the patient will not have any lasting damage. Most seizures are have no known cause and are referred to as epilepsy.

T3 SIMULATION SYSTEM

Seizure: Performance

Performance Checklist **Role:** **Start Time:** **End Time:**

Expected Actions	Time	2	1	0	N/A
1. Scene Size-up *					
2. PS: CC, LOC					
3. PS: ABCs					
4. Intervention: Airway monitoring , 100% 02 BVM *					
5. SA: Vitals and Monitor					
6. SA: Blood Sugar					
7. Intervention: Switch NRB					
8. Past Medical History					
9. Differential Diagnosis *					
10. IV Access					
11. Transport: Non-emergent					
12. Reassessment					
13. Medication - Versed *					
14. Report					
(*) actions are Mandatory					
TEAMWORK/LEADERSHIP					
1. Coordination					
2. Flexibility					
3. Communication - CLC					
4. Affect - Possible refusal, Reassurance *					
5. Overall					

SELF EVALUATION: ☐ Successful ☐ Unsuccessful **SCORE:** /38

NOTES:

Potentially Harmful/ Dangerous Actions (omission, commission, sequencing):

C DEBRIEFING

Debriefing Questions:

1. How did feel throughout the simulation experience?
2. What were your primary diagnoses in this scenario?
3. Did you feel you had the knowledge and skills to care for this patient? Why/ why not?
4. What were your priority assessments and interventions?
5. What outcomes did you measure?
6. What did you do well?
7. What was missed? What would you have done differently?
8. Is there anything else you would like to discuss?

Critical Thinking

1. What is your immediate priority with this patient?

2. Is determining the cause of the seizure important?

3. How serious is this patient?

4. What is the most common cause of seizures?

5. What is the ALS treatment for status seizures?

6. What are the warnings and side effects of this drug?

T3 SIMULATION SYSTEM

Seizure: Performance

Performance Checklist Role: | Start Time: End Time:

Expected Actions	Time	2	1	0	N/A
1. Scene Size-up *					
2. PS: CC, LOC					
3. PS: ABCs					
4. Intervention: Airway monitoring , 100% 02 BVM					
5. SA: Vitals and Monitor					
6. SA: Blood Sugar -22*					
7. Differential Diagnosis *: Hypoglycemia					
8. TI: IV access*					
9. TI: 25mg Glucose*					
10. Reassessment					
11. Transport: Non-emergent					
12. Reassessment					
13. Report					
(*) actions are Mandatory					
TEAMWORK/LEADERSHIP					
1. Coordination					
2. Flexibility					
3. Communication - CLC					
4. Affect - Possible refusal, Reassurance *					
5. Overall					

SELF EVALUATION: ☐ Successful ☐ Unsuccessful | **SCORE:** /36

NOTES:

Potentially Harmful/ Dangerous Actions (omission, commission, sequencing):

C DEBRIEFING

Debriefing Questions:

1. How did feel throughout the simulation experience?
2. What were your primary diagnoses in this scenario?
3. Did you feel you had the knowledge and skills to care for this patient? Why/ why not?
4. What were your priority assessments and interventions?
5. What outcomes did you measure?
6. What did you do well?
7. What was missed? What would you have done differently?
8. Is there anything else you would like to discuss?

Critical Thinking

1. What treatment and concerns do you have during transport?

2. Do all seizure patients need to be transported to the ED or can they stay home with a call to their neurologist?

3. Distinguish between a provoked seizure and epilepsy.

EMS PATIENT CARE REPORT (PCR) Scenario:

PATIENT INFORMATION

Name: Age: Sex: Weight: Kg (lb)	Allergies: Medications: Past Medical History: Chief Complaint:

VITAL SIGNS

Time:	BP:	Pulse:	Respiration:	Sao_2:
Time:	BP:	Pulse:	Respiration:	Sao_2:
Time:	BP:	Pulse:	Respiration:	Sao_2:

PHYSICAL / NEUROLOGICAL EXAM

LOC: Oriented: GCS: Pupils: Sensory/Motor: Facial Droop: Speech:	Skin: HEENT: Neck: Chest: Respiratory: Cardiovascular: EKG:	AB/GI: Pelvis: GU: Posterior : Extremities: Psychiatric: GLU:

CHIEF COMPLAINT

HISTORY OF PRESENT ILLNESS

NOTES

EMS PATIENT CARE REPORT (PCR) Scenario:

PATIENT INFORMATION

Name:	Allergies:
Age:	Medications:
Sex:	Past Medical History:
Weight: Kg (lb)	Chief Complaint:

VITAL SIGNS

Time:	BP:	Pulse:	Respiration:	Sao_2:
Time:	BP:	Pulse:	Respiration:	Sao_2:
Time:	BP:	Pulse:	Respiration:	Sao_2:

PHYSICAL / NEUROLOGICAL EXAM

LOC:	Skin:	AB/GI:
Oriented:	HEENT:	Pelvis:
GCS:	Neck:	GU:
Pupils:	Chest:	Posterior :
Sensory/Motor:	Respiratory:	Extremities:
Facial Droop:	Cardiovascular:	Psychiatric:
Speech:	EKG:	GLU:

CHIEF COMPLAINT

HISTORY OF PRESENT ILLNESS

NOTES

ADULT TRAUMA SOFT TISSUE BURNS

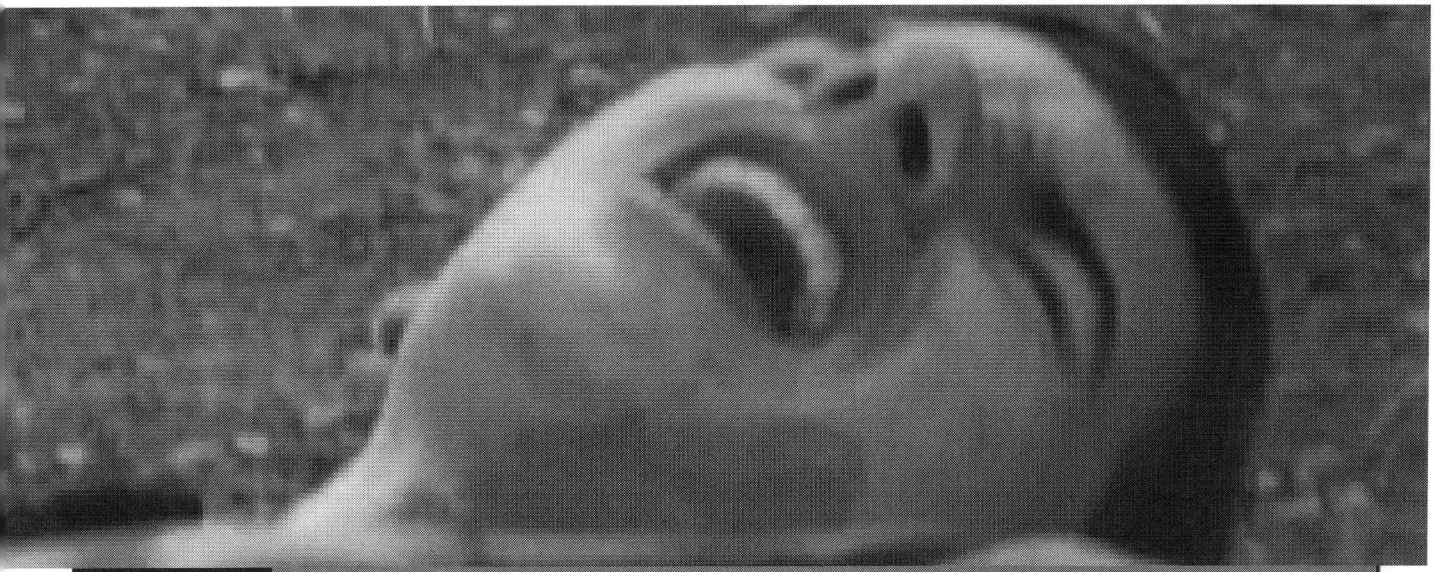

21 Y/O MALE, EXTENSIVE UPPER BODY BURNS

DISPATCH
Location: Farm yard
Type of situation: Severe burns
Number of patients: 1
Hazards: Active fire ground

OBJECTIVES

1. Assessment of scene safety.
2. Assessment of the burned patient (BSA)
3. Understand the pathophysiology of burns.
4. Prioritize interventions
5. Perform appropriate interventions.
6. Demonstrate effective teamwork.

SCENE SIZE-UP	
OVERALL SAFETY	ACTIVE FIREGROUND
MOI / NOI	GAS EXPLOSION, EXTENSIVE UPPER BODY BURNS
RESOURCES	BLS RESPONSE
C-SPINE	POSSIBLE TRAUMA

PATHOPHYSIOLOGY

Overview Scenario 1 :

Burns disrupt or destroy the body's protective barrier to the outside environment. The extent and depth of the burn will determine the severity. Burns are now classified as superficial, partial or full thickness. While it is important to determine the total body surface area that is burned, it is not critical to determine whether it is partial or full thickness.

All burned patients must be evaluated for airway injury and smoke inhalation. Early management of a possible airway injury and smoke inhalation is essential. Any disruption of normal speech (phonation), secretions that have soot, difficulty breathing, being trapped in a closed space fire and any loss of consciousness while in a fire are indicators of airway injury.

Treatment for burns are to manage any airway injuries, prevent further injury by removing any heat sources, cover the burned area with a clean, dry sheet, provide fluid resuscitation , provide adequate pain relief, prevent hypothermia, and transport to the appropriate facility.

Overview Scenario 2:

Electrical burns cause injury 3 different methods: 1) Cardiac Arrest due to the electrical effects on the heart, 2) Muscle, nerve and tissue destruction from the electrical current passing through the body, 3) Contact thermal burns at entry and exit site.
Tissue damage is dependent upon the length of time in contact with the source, and the type and strength of the voltage. The electricity travels through the body along the path of least resistance, nerves muscles, and blood vessels. These will be injured in a serious electrical burn.

Electrical burns are either low tension (less than 500 volts) or high tension (greater than 500 volts). Low tension are often small burns at the source of contact but may be full thickness usually from the arc or flash that can reach 4000°C.
High tension will have an entrance and an exit and may have significant internal injuries including coagulation necrosis and compartment syndrome. Cardiac arrhythmias are also common with high tension burns. Ventricular arrhythmias, ventricular standstill and respiratory paralysis are all seen with high voltage contact.

Treatment is supportive, ACLS for cardiac arrest, and cardiac arrhythmias, intubation and BVM for respiratory paralysis. IV access in a non-burned site, with a fluid bolus of 10-20 ml/kg NS for hypotension. Dress and bandage external burns, treat for pain, and monitor all vital signs frequently. Protect C-Spine since many patients get thrown from DC wires upon contact. Keep patient warm. Scene safety is paramount, as the current can arc up to 30 feet from an energized wire.

Scene safety is paramount, as the current can arc up to 30 feet from an energized wire.

Soft Tissue Burn: Performance

Performance Checklist Role:

Start Time:	End Time:

Expected Actions	Time	2	1	0	N/A
1. Scene Size up *					
2. Remove burning clothing*					
3. Primary Survey					
4. TI: Apply 100% O2 NRB					
5. Secondary Assessment					
6. SA: BSA estimate: 36%*					
7. D DX: Life threatening burns*					
8. TI: Pain Meds - IN*					
9. Immobilization and evacuation to warm ambulance.*					
10. Reassessment					
11. TI: Humidified 02 & nebulizer					
12. TI: IV access & fluids*					
13. Contact Med Control for Fluid rate.					
14.IV pain & Solumedrol*					
15. Reassesment w distal pulses.					
16. Report					
TEAMWORK/LEADERSHIP					
1. Coordination					
2. Flexibility					
3. Communication					
4. Affect: Rapport & Support*					
5. Overall					

*actions are mandatory

SELF EVALUATION: ☐ **Successful** ☐ **Unsuccessful**

SCORE: /42

NOTES:

Potentially Harmful/ Dangerous Actions (omission, commission, sequencing):

C DEBRIEFING

Debriefing Questions:

1. How did you feel throughout the simulation experience?
2. What were your primary diagnoses in this scenario?
3. What was the total burn area?

   Arms= 18%, Thorax=18 %, Some neck TBSA= +/- 36 %
4. Did you feel you had the knowledge and skills to care for this patient? Why/ why not?
5. What were your priority assessments and interventions?
6. Why is it so important to get the patient to the ambulance immediately?
7. What outcomes did you measure?
8. What did you do well?
9. What was missed? What would you have done differently?

Critical Thinking

10. What is the importance of checking distal pulses repeatedly?
11. What is compartment syndrome and how does that relate to this patient.
12. Is there anything else you would like to discuss?

T3 SIMULATION SYSTEM

Electrical Burn: Performance

Performance Checklist Role: | Start Time: | End Time:

Expected Actions	Time	2	1	0	N/A
1.Scene Safety / Transport Decision*					
2. CSpine					
3. Primary Survey					
4. O2/ BVM*					
5.Secondary Assessment.					
6. Dress wounds					
7. Affect: Communicate with Family*					
8 Immobilize and Extricate					
9. Reassessment					
10. 12 lead EKG*					
11 TI: Transcutaneous Pacing*					
12. TI: Medications*					
13. Report					
TEAMWORK/LEADERSHIP					
1. Coordination					
2. Flexibility					
3. Communication					
4. Affect: Rapport & Support*					
5. Overall					

* Actions are mandatory

SELF EVALUATION: ☐ **Successful** ☐ **Unsuccessful**

SCORE: /36

NOTES:

Potentially Harmful/Dangerous Actions (omission, commission, sequencing):

C DEBRIEFING

Debriefing Questions:

1. How did you feel throughout the simulation experience?
2. What were your primary diagnoses in this scenario?
3. Did you feel you had the knowledge and skills to care for this patient? Why/ why not?
3. What were your priority assessments and interventions?
4. What outcomes did you measure?
5. What did you do well?
6. What was missed? What would you have done differently?

Critical Thinking

7. What are the common arrhythmias with a high tension burn? (Ventricular)
8. How serious do you think the internal injures will be? (Serious)
9. Why should you look for and entrance and exit wound. (There may be extensive burns and injuries)
10. Why is it important to check distal pulse frequently? (frequent compartment syndrome with electrical burns)
11. What is compartment syndrome and how does that relate to this patient.

EMS PATIENT CARE REPORT (PCR) Scenario:

PATIENT INFORMATION

Name:	Allergies:
Age:	Medications:
Sex:	Past Medical History:
Weight: Kg (lb)	Chief Complaint:

VITAL SIGNS

Time:	BP:	Pulse:	Respiration:	Sao_2:
Time:	BP:	Pulse:	Respiration:	Sao_2:
Time:	BP:	Pulse:	Respiration:	Sao_2:

PHYSICAL / NEUROLOGICAL EXAM

LOC:	Skin:	AB/GI:
Oriented:	HEENT:	Pelvis:
GCS:	Neck:	GU:
Pupils:	Chest:	Posterior :
Sensory/Motor:	Respiratory:	Extremities:
Facial Droop:	Cardiovascular:	Psychiatric:
Speech:	EKG:	GLU:

CHIEF COMPLAINT

HISTORY OF PRESENT ILLNESS

NOTES

EMS PATIENT CARE REPORT (PCR) Scenario:

PATIENT INFORMATION

Name:	Allergies:
Age:	Medications:
Sex:	Past Medical History:
Weight: Kg (lb)	Chief Complaint:

VITAL SIGNS

Time:	BP:	Pulse:	Respiration:	Sao_2:
Time:	BP:	Pulse:	Respiration:	Sao_2:
Time:	BP:	Pulse:	Respiration:	Sao_2:

PHYSICAL / NEUROLOGICAL EXAM

LOC:	Skin:	AB/GI:
Oriented:	HEENT:	Pelvis:
GCS:	Neck:	GU:
Pupils:	Chest:	Posterior :
Sensory/Motor:	Respiratory:	Extremities:
Facial Droop:	Cardiovascular:	Psychiatric:
Speech:	EKG:	GLU:

CHIEF COMPLAINT

HISTORY OF PRESENT ILLNESS

NOTES

ADULT TRAUMA HEAD INJURY

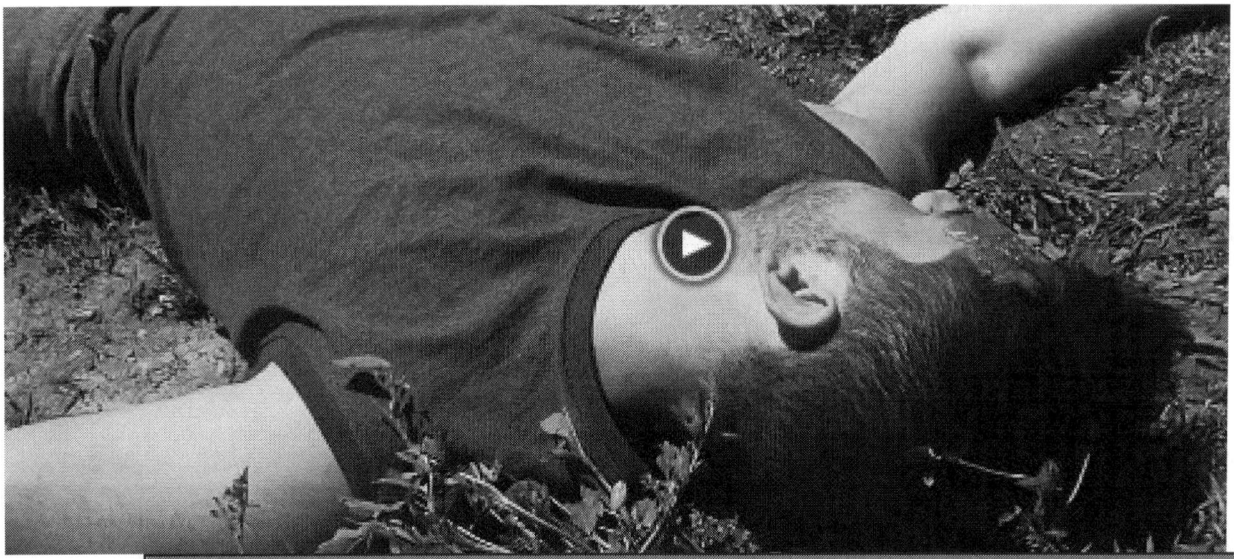

21 Y/O MALE, HEAD INJURY AFTER ATV CRASH

DISPATCH
Location: Rural trail
Number of patients: 1
Type of situation:Head injury, ATV crash
Hazards: Unknown
Hospitals: Regional Hospital 20 minutes, Level 1 Trauma 50 minutes

OBJECTIVES

a. Assessment of the patient
b. Prioritize interventions
c. Recognition of head injury
d. Perform correct and timely interventions - airway mngt
e. Appropriate transport decision
f. Demonstrate effective teamwork

SCENE SIZE-UP	
OVERALL SAFETY	UNKNOWN
MOI / NOI	ALTERED MENTAL STATUS, HEAD INJURY AFTER ATV CRASH, EXTENSIVE DAMAGE ATV
RESOURCES	BLS RESPONSE, FD DISPATCHED
C-SPINE	POSSIBLE TRAUMA

PATHOPHYSIOLOGY

Overview:

Head Injury with swelling due to injury or bleeding will create a cycle of events that can cause rapid deterioration. In the event of an epidural bleed, the patient may experience unconsciousness after the injury, awaking to a lucid interval, and then rapid deterioration. Epidural bleeds are arterial causing a rapid increase in intercranial pressure. As the pressure increases the body increases blood pressure to try to perfuse the brain. The pressure in the skull begins to herniated the brain which puts pressure on the vagus nerve and slows the heart. Signs include increasing BP, slowing heart rate and irregular or apneic breathing. Slower bleeds can produce neurological deficits and may present with symptoms hours to days later. Treatment is transport to a trauma hospital . Internal structural damage inside the skull is likely with unequal pupil response and/or dilation. Signs of herniation are defined by Cushings Triad.

Blunt Head Injury: Performance

Performance Checklist | **Role:** | **Start Time:** **End Time:**

Expected Actions	Time	2	1	0	N/A
1. Scene Safety*					
2. Spinal immobilization*					
3. Transport decision*					
4. Primary Survey					
5. Secondary assessment					
6. D DX: Epidural bleed*					
7. TI: Splint ankle					
8. TI: Immobilize / Extricate					
9. Transport: Emergent					
10. Reassessment					
11. TI: BVM*					
12. TI: IV access and fluids*					
13. TI: RSI Meds*					
14. TI: Intubate*					
15. Reassessment					
16. Report					
TEAMWORK/LEADERSHIP					
1. Coordination*					
2. Flexibility					
3. Communication					
4. Affect: Rapport & Support					
5. Overall					

*Actions are mandatory

SELF EVALUATION: ☐ **Successful** ☐ **Unsuccessful** | **SCORE: /42**

NOTES:

Potentially Harmful/Dangerous Actions (omission, commission, sequencing):

C DEBRIEFING

Debriefing Questions:

1. How did you feel throughout the simulation experience?
2. What were your priority assessments and interventions?
3. What did you do well?
4. What was missed? What would you have done differently?
5. Is there anything else you would like to discuss?

Critical Thinking

1. What is the problem with this patient?
2. How serious is it?
3. What is the most important field care?
4. What is the rationale for RSI?

T3 SIMULATION SYSTEM

Blunt Head Injury: Performance

Performance Checklist **Role:** **Start Time:** **End Time:**

Expected Actions	Time	2	1	0	N/A
1. Scene Safety*					
2. Spinal immobilization*					
3. Transport decision					
4. Primary Survey					
5. Secondary assessment					
6. D DX:*					
7. TI:					
8. Transport					
9. Reassessment					
10. TI:					
11. TI:					
12. TI:					
13. TI:					
14. Reassessment					
15. Report					
TEAMWORK/LEADERSHIP					
1. Coordination					
2. Flexibility					
3. Communication					
4. Affect: Rapport & Support					
5. Overall					

* Actions are mandatory

SELF EVALUATION: ☐ **Successful** ☐ **Unsuccessful**

SCORE: /40

NOTES:

Potentially Harmful/Dangerous Actions (omission, commission, sequencing):

C DEBRIEFING

Debriefing Questions:

1. How did you feel throughout the simulation experience?

2. What were your priority assessments and interventions?

3. What did you do well?

4. What was missed? What would you have done differently?

5. Is there anything else you would like to discuss?

Critical Thinking

1. What is the problem with this patient?

2. How serious is it?

3. What is the most important field care?

EMS PATIENT CARE REPORT (PCR) Scenario:

PATIENT INFORMATION

Name:	Allergies:
Age:	Medications:
Sex:	Past Medical History:
Weight: Kg (lb)	Chief Complaint:

VITAL SIGNS

Time:	BP:	Pulse:	Respiration:	Sao_2:
Time:	BP:	Pulse:	Respiration:	Sao_2:
Time:	BP:	Pulse:	Respiration:	Sao_2:

PHYSICAL / NEUROLOGICAL EXAM

LOC:	Skin:	AB/GI:
Oriented:	HEENT:	Pelvis:
GCS:	Neck:	GU:
Pupils:	Chest:	Posterior :
Sensory/Motor:	Respiratory:	Extremities:
Facial Droop:	Cardiovascular:	Psychiatric:
Speech:	EKG:	GLU:

CHIEF COMPLAINT

HISTORY OF PRESENT ILLNESS

NOTES

EMS PATIENT CARE REPORT (PCR) Scenario:

PATIENT INFORMATION

Name:
Age:
Sex:
Weight: Kg (lb)

Allergies:
Medications:
Past Medical History:
Chief Complaint:

VITAL SIGNS

Time:	BP:	Pulse:	Respiration:	Sao_2:
Time:	BP:	Pulse:	Respiration:	Sao_2:
Time:	BP:	Pulse:	Respiration:	Sao_2:

PHYSICAL / NEUROLOGICAL EXAM

LOC:
Oriented:
GCS:
Pupils:
Sensory/Motor:
Facial Droop:
Speech:

Skin:
HEENT:
Neck:
Chest:
Respiratory:
Cardiovascular:
EKG:

AB/GI:
Pelvis:
GU:
Posterior :
Extremities:
Psychiatric:
GLU:

CHIEF COMPLAINT

HISTORY OF PRESENT ILLNESS

NOTES

ADULT HEAT EMERGENCY

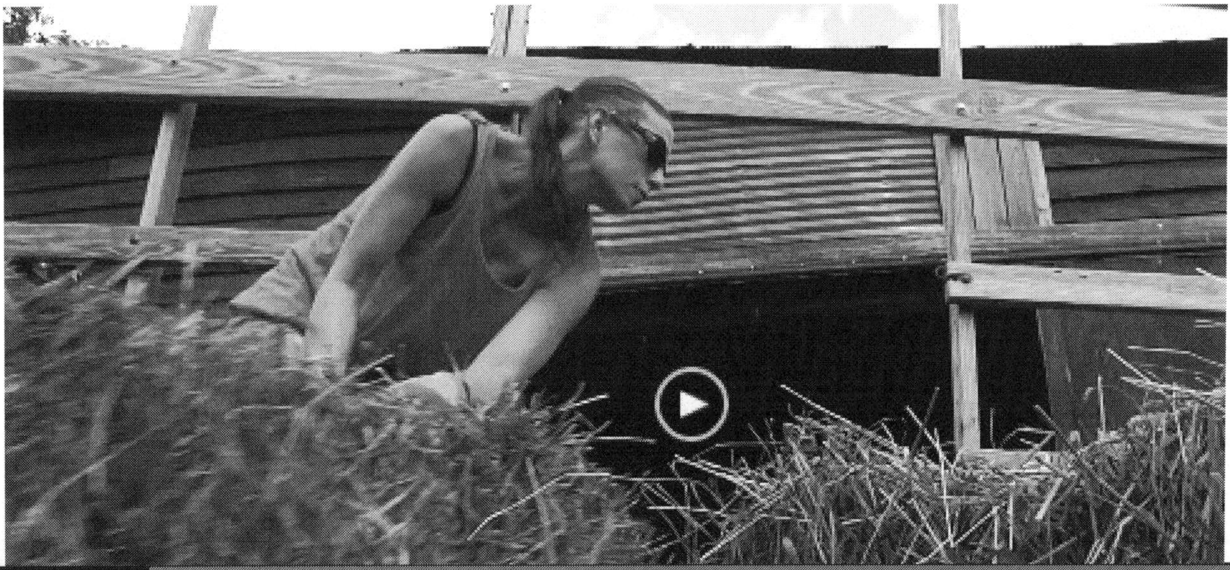

36 Y/O FEMALE, OVERHEATED, STOMACH CRAMPS

DISPATCH
Location: Rural farm
Type of situation: Overheated, stomach cramps
Number of patients: 1
Hazards: No hazards, heatwave

OBJECTIVES
1. Assessment of the scene and the patient.
2. Understand the pathophysiology of a heat emergency.
3. Recognize the symptoms of heat cramps, heat exhaustion, and heat stroke.
4. Prioritize and perform appropriate interventions- (cooling the patient, oral fluid replacement)
5. Demonstrate effective teamwork

SCENE SIZE-UP	
OVERALL SAFETY	SCENE IS SAFE
MOI / NOI	OVERHEATED with STOMACH CRAMPS
RESOURCES	BLS RESPONSE
C-SPINE	NO SIGNS OF TRAUMA

PATHOPHYSIOLOGY

Overview:

Heat emergencies constitute a continuum from heat cramps to heat exhaustion to heat stroke.

Heat cramps are the result of loss of essential fluids (water) and electrolytes. The result is spasms and cramps of the large muscle groups (legs, abdominal, and back).

As the loss of water and electrolytes continues heat exhaustion may occur. Heat exhaustion may present with an altered level of consciousness such as dizziness, fainting, and weakness. Sweating should also be present, but sweating may not be effective due to fluid loss, humidity, or clothing. The patient's core temperature is normal or slightly elevated.

If the patient's ability to sweat becomes impaired and the body's thermo-regulatory mechanism is lost, a life threating condition called heat stroke may occur. It is characterized by very hot and pale/ashen skin.

SIMULATION SYSTEM

Heat Emergency: Performance

Performance Checklist Role: | Start Time: End Time:

Expected Actions	Time	2	1	0	N/A
1. Scene size-up *					
2. PS: CC, LOC, HPI					
3. PS: ABCs, 100% O2 NC					
4. TI: Active cooling *					
5. Transport: Cool ambulance *					
6. SA: Vital signs					
7 TI: Provide Oral fluid *					
8. Rapid cooling *					
9. DD: Heat Exhaustion *					
10. IV fluid replacement Zofran if nausea/vomiting *					
11. SA: 12 lead EKG					
12. SA: Blood sugar					
13. Report *					
TEAMWORK/LEADERSHIP					
1. Coordination					
2. Flexibility					
3. Communication					
4.Affect: Rapport and Support					
5. Overall					

(*) Actions are mandatory

SELF EVALUATION: ☐ **Successful** ☐ **Unsuccessful** | **SCORE: /36**

NOTES:

Potentially Harmful/Dangerous actions (omission, commission, sequencing):

C DEBRIEFING

Debriefing Questions:

1. How did feel throughout the simulation experience?

2. What were your primary diagnoses in this scenario?

3. Did you feel you had the knowledge and skills to care for this patient? Why/ why not?

4. What were your priority assessments and interventions?

5. What outcomes did you measure?

6. What did you do well?

7. What was missed? What would you have done differently?

Critical Thinking

1. What is the priority in heat exhaustion vs. heat stroke?

2. Who is likely to get heat exhaustion?

3. How aggressive should treatment for heat stroke be?

T3 SIMULATION SYSTEM

Heat Emergency: Performance

Performance Checklist Role: | Start Time: End Time:

Expected Actions	Time	2	1	0	N/A
1. Scene size-up *					
2. PS: CC, LOC, HPI					
3. PS: ABCs, 100% O2 NC					
4. TI: Active cooling *					
5. Transport: Cool ambulance *					
6. SA: Vital signs					
7 TI: Provide Oral fluid *					
8. Rapid cooling *					
9. DD: Heat Exhaustion *					
10. IV fluid replacement					
Zofran if nausea/vomiting *					
11. SA: 12 lead EKG					
12. SA: Blood sugar					
13. Report *					
TEAMWORK/LEADERSHIP					
1. Coordination					
2. Flexibility					
3. Communication					
4.Affect: Rapport and Support					
5. Overall					

(*) Actions are mandatory

SELF EVALUATION: ☐ Successful ☐ Unsuccessful

SCORE: /36

NOTES:

Potentially Harmful/Dangerous actions (omission, commission, sequencing):

C DEBRIEFING

Debriefing Questions:

1. How did feel throughout the simulation experience?

2. What were your primary diagnoses in this scenario?

3. Did you feel you had the knowledge and skills to care for this patient? Why/ why not?

4. What were your priority assessments and interventions?

5. What outcomes did you measure?

6. What did you do well?

7. What was missed? What would you have done differently?

Critical Thinking

1. Who is likely to get heat stroke?

EMS PATIENT CARE REPORT (PCR) Scenario:

PATIENT INFORMATION

Name:	Allergies:
Age:	Medications:
Sex:	Past Medical History:
Weight: Kg (lb)	Chief Complaint:

VITAL SIGNS

Time:	BP:	Pulse:	Respiration:	Sao_2:
Time:	BP:	Pulse:	Respiration:	Sao_2:
Time:	BP:	Pulse:	Respiration:	Sao_2:

PHYSICAL / NEUROLOGICAL EXAM

LOC:	Skin:	AB/GI:
Oriented:	HEENT:	Pelvis:
GCS:	Neck:	GU:
Pupils:	Chest:	Posterior :
Sensory/Motor:	Respiratory:	Extremities:
Facial Droop:	Cardiovascular:	Psychiatric:
Speech:	EKG:	GLU:

CHIEF COMPLAINT

HISTORY OF PRESENT ILLNESS

NOTES

EMS PATIENT CARE REPORT (PCR) Scenario:

PATIENT INFORMATION

Name:	Allergies:
Age:	Medications:
Sex:	Past Medical History:
Weight: Kg (lb)	Chief Complaint:

VITAL SIGNS

Time:	BP:	Pulse:	Respiration:	Sao_2:
Time:	BP:	Pulse:	Respiration:	Sao_2:
Time:	BP:	Pulse:	Respiration:	Sao_2:

PHYSICAL / NEUROLOGICAL EXAM

LOC:	Skin:	AB/GI:
Oriented:	HEENT:	Pelvis:
GCS:	Neck:	GU:
Pupils:	Chest:	Posterior :
Sensory/Motor:	Respiratory:	Extremities:
Facial Droop:	Cardiovascular:	Psychiatric:
Speech:	EKG:	GLU:

CHIEF COMPLAINT

HISTORY OF PRESENT ILLNESS

NOTES

ADULT TRAUMA MULTI-SYSTEM

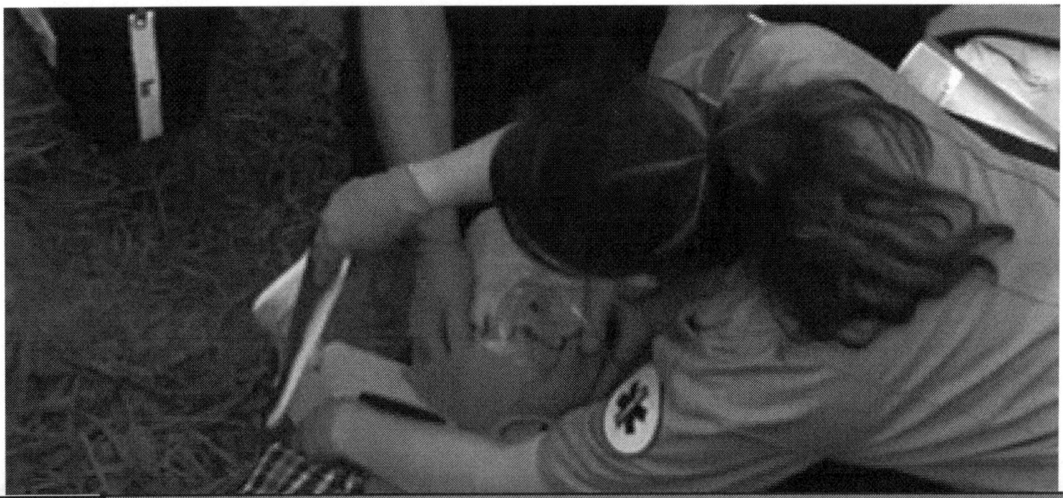

46 Y/O MALE, CRUSH VICTIM TRACTOR ROLLOVER

DISPATCH

Location: Farm field

Number of patients: 1

Type of situation: Crushed patient

Hazards: Unknown

OBJECTIVES

a. Assessment of the patient.
b. Understanding of the pathophysiology of multisystem trauma.
c. Recognition of the signs, symptoms and circumstances that can result from crush injuries.
d. Recognition of the signs, symptoms of internal bleeding.
e. Performance of appropriate interventions.
f. Demonstration of effective teamwork with all responders.

SCENE SIZE-UP	
OVERALL SAFETY	SCENE SAFETY UNKNOWN
MOI / NOI	TRACTOR ROLLOVER
RESOURCES	ALS RESPONSE
C-SPINE	SIGNS OF TRAUMA

PATHOPHYSIOLOGY

Overview:

Crush injuries can result in the release of toxins into the blood stream upon extrication including life threating levels of potassium. Other toxins that are released from dying muscle are myoglobin, calcium, and lactic acid. These toxins may result in kidney damage or death, and ventricular arrhythmias. Compartment syndrome of the trapped area or any area distal to the injury is likely. Extraction of the patient from the object may have to be delayed until proper evaluation and treatment has been initiated.

Treatment must begin prior to extrication. Early contact with the Regional Trauma Center is essential; a physician may be needed at the scene. Early fluid resuscitation is indicated. ALS evaluation of hyperkalemia must occur prior, during, and post extrication. Sodium Bicarbonate may be required to prevent cardiac arrhythmias from hyperkalemia. Treatment for a cardiac arrest secondary to hyperkalemia includes Sodium Bicarbonate,-

Calcium Chloride, and Albuterol.

Trauma - Multisystem Performance

Performance Checklist Role:

Start Time: **End Time:**

Expected Actions	Time	2	1	0	N/A
1. Scene Safety*					
2. Primary Survey					
3. O2 100% NRB					
4. SA: Monitor*					
5. Differential Dx: Hyperkalemia, Crush injury*					
5. TI: Pre-treat medications*					
6. IV access X 2*					
7. Coordinate lift with medical control, Medevac and FD*					
8. TI: Bicarb, calcium on release*					
9. TI: Pelvic sling*					
10, TI: Scoop stretcher					
11. Reassessment					
12. Albuterol					
13. Communication: Summary					
TEAMWORK/LEADERSHIP					
1. Coordination					
2. Flexibility					
3. Communication					
4. Affect: Rapport & Support					
5. Overall					

*actions are mandatory

SELF EVALUATION: ☐ Successful ☐ Unsuccessful

SCORE:

NOTES:

Potentially Harmful/ Dangerous Actions (omission, commission, sequencing):

C DEBRIEFING

10. Debriefing Questions:

1. How did you feel throughout the simulation experience?
2. What were your primary diagnoses in this scenario?
3. Did you feel you had the knowledge and skills to care for this patient? Why/ why not?
4. What were your priority assessments and interventions?
5. What outcomes did you measure?
6. What did you do well?
7. What was missed? What would you have done differently?
8. Is there anything else you would like to discuss?

11. Critical Thinking

1. Why is the time frame for extrication important?

2. Is taking time to put pelvic sling on necessary?

3. Is it possible to bleed to death from this injury?

Trauma - Multisystem Performance

Performance | Role: | Start Time: | End Time:

Expected Actions	Time	2	1	0	N/A
1. Scene Safety*					
2. Primary Survey					
3. O2 100% NRB					
4. SA: Monitor*					
5. Differential Dx: Hyperkalemia, Crush injury*					
5. TI: Pre-treat medications*					
6. IV access X 2*					
7. Coordinate lift *					
8. TI: Bicarb, calcium on release*					
9. TI: Pelvic sling*					
10, TI: Scoop stretcher					
11. Reassessment					
12. Albuterol					
13. Communication: Summary					
TEAMWORK/LEADERSHIP					
1. Coordination					
2. Flexibility					
3. Communication					
4. Affect: Rapport & Support					
5. Overall					

* actions are mandatory

SELF EVALUATION: ☐ Successful ☐ Unsuccessful

SCORE:

NOTES:

Potentially Harmful/ Dangerous Actions (omission, commission, sequencing):

C DEBRIEFING

10. Debriefing Questions:

1. How did you feel throughout the simulation experience?
2. What were your primary diagnoses in this scenario?
3. Did you feel you had the knowledge and skills to care for this patient? Why/ why not?
4. What were your priority assessments and interventions?
5. What outcomes did you measure?
6. What did you do well?
7. What was missed? What would you have done differently?
8. Is there anything else you would like to discuss?

Critical Thinking

1. Describe the prehospital management of crush injuries.

EMS PATIENT CARE REPORT (PCR) Scenario:

PATIENT INFORMATION

Name:	Allergies:
Age:	Medications:
Sex:	Past Medical History:
Weight: Kg (lb)	Chief Complaint:

VITAL SIGNS

Time:	BP:	Pulse:	Respiration:	Sao_2:
Time:	BP:	Pulse:	Respiration:	Sao_2:
Time:	BP:	Pulse:	Respiration:	Sao_2:

PHYSICAL / NEUROLOGICAL EXAM

LOC:	Skin:	AB/GI:
Oriented:	HEENT:	Pelvis:
GCS:	Neck:	GU:
Pupils:	Chest:	Posterior :
Sensory/Motor:	Respiratory:	Extremities:
Facial Droop:	Cardiovascular:	Psychiatric:
Speech:	EKG:	GLU:

CHIEF COMPLAINT

HISTORY OF PRESENT ILLNESS

NOTES

EMS PATIENT CARE REPORT (PCR) Scenario:

PATIENT INFORMATION

Name: Age: Sex: Weight: Kg (lb)	Allergies: Medications: Past Medical History: Chief Complaint:

VITAL SIGNS

Time:	BP:	Pulse:	Respiration:	Sao_2:
Time:	BP:	Pulse:	Respiration:	Sao_2:
Time:	BP:	Pulse:	Respiration:	Sao_2:

PHYSICAL / NEUROLOGICAL EXAM

LOC:	Skin:	AB/GI:
Oriented:	HEENT:	Pelvis:
GCS:	Neck:	GU:
Pupils:	Chest:	Posterior :
Sensory/Motor:	Respiratory:	Extremities:
Facial Droop:	Cardiovascular:	Psychiatric:
Speech:	EKG:	GLU:

CHIEF COMPLAINT

HISTORY OF PRESENT ILLNESS

NOTES

ADULT TRAUMA PARTIAL AMPUTATION

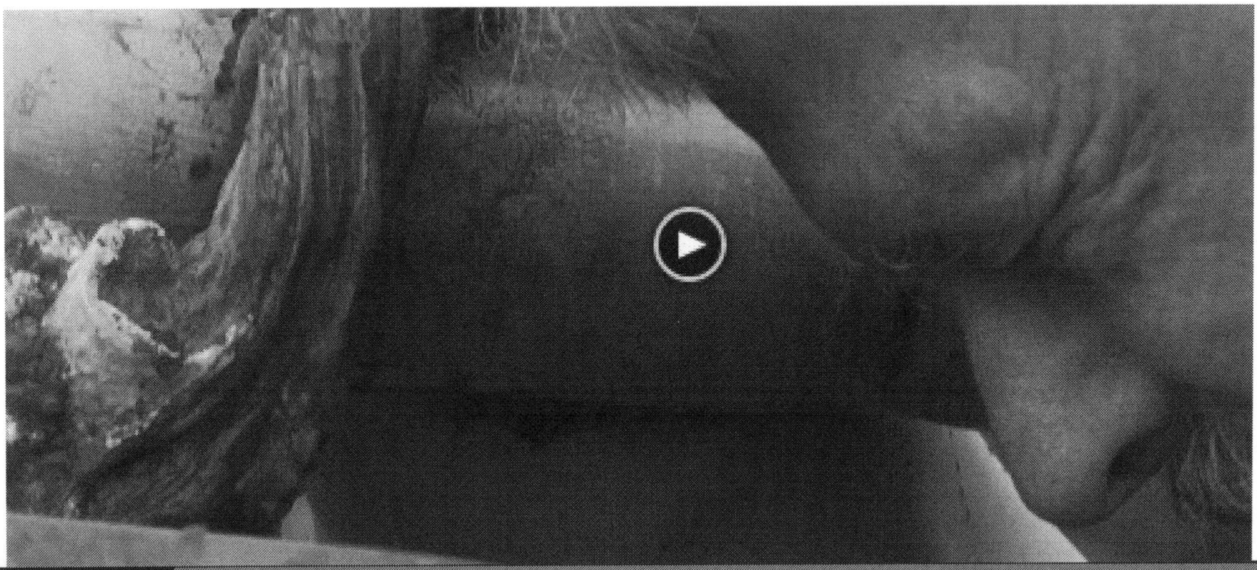

55 Y/O MALE, PARTIAL AMPUTATION, EXTREMITY ENTANGLEMENT

DISPATCH
Location: Dairy farm
Type of situation:Partial amputation, trauma
Number of patients: 1
Hazards: Unknown

OBJECTIVES
1. Assessment of the scene and the patient.
2. Recognize need for immediate bleeding control
3. Prioritization and performance of appropriate interventions
4. Recognition of signs and symptoms of shock
5. Recognize need for immediate transport
6. Demonstration of effective teamwork.

SCENE SIZE-UP	
OVERALL SAFETY	FD HAS ALSO BEEN DISPATCHED, TRACTOR STILL RUNNING
MOI / NOI	EXTREMITY ENTANGLEMENT, PARTIAL AMPUTATION, SHOCK
RESOURCES	BLS RESPONSE
C-SPINE	SIGNS OF TRAUMA. PTOs ROTATE AT EXTREMELY HIGH RPM.

PATHOPHYSIOLOGY

Overview:

A trapped extremity results in dual expectations. The primary expectation is for the survivability of the patient. The second is the salvagability of the extremity.

Treatment must begin prior to removal of the entrapped extremity. If the extremity has been trapped for longer than 2 hours, the responder must begin treatment for crush injury. Toxins leaking from the injured tissue can cause serious renal and cardiac problems. If these toxins accumulate in the damaged limb then are released into the central circulation en mass, elevated blood levels of potassium, myoglobin, and lactic acid will occur. The result may be cardiac arrhythmias, end organ failure or even cardiac arrest.

Compartment syndrome occurs when edema from the damaged muscle causes restriction of blood flow to that muscle. This results in muscle death if blood flow is not restored.

In addition, pain and anxiety management are essential while the limb is being extricated. Lengthy and difficult extrications may require a physician to come to the scene for advanced care.

To preserve the limb it is necessary to limit additional damage, restore blood flow and anatomical position if possible, and select the hospital destination.

T3 SIMULATION SYSTEM

Partial Amputation

Performance Checklist Role: **Start Time:** **End Time:**

Expected Actions	Time	2	1	0	N/A
1. SSU: lock out- tag out*					
2. TI: Tourniquet*					
3. Primary Survey					
4. TI: O2 100% NRB					
5. SA: Vitals					
6. TI: IV access*					
7. TI: Fluid bolus*					
8. Splint wound*					
9. Immobilize and extricate*					
10. Reassessment					
11. TI: Pain meds					
12. Transport: Emergent					
13. Reassessment					
14. TI: 2nd tourniquet*					
15. SA: head to toe exam					
16. Reassessment					
17. Report					
TEAMWORK/LEADERSHIP					
1. Coordination					
2. Flexibility					
3. Communication					
4. Affect: Rapport & Support					
5. Overall					

RED Actions are mandatory.

SELF EVALUATION: ☐ **Successful** ☐ **Unsuccessful**

SCORE: /44

NOTES:

Potentially Harmful/Dangerous actions (omission, commission, sequencing):

Partial Amputation: Debriefing

C DEBRIEFING

Debriefing Questions:

1. How did you feel throughout the simulation experience?
2. What were your primary diagnoses in this scenario?
3. Did you feel you had the knowledge and skills to care for this patient? Why/ why not?
4. What were your priority assessments and interventions?
5. What outcomes did you measure?
6. What did you do well?
7. What was missed? What would you have done differently?
8. Is there anything else you would like to discuss?

Critical Thinking

1. Why is the time frame for extrication important?
2. Where the tourniquet should be placed? What artery is located there?
3. Is this arm salvageable?
4. Is it possible to bleed to death from this injury?

Partial Amputation

Performance Checklist | Role: | Start Time: | End Time:

Expected Actions	Time	2	1	0	N/A
1. SSU: lock out- tag out*					
2. TI: Tourniquet*					
3. Primary Survey					
4. TI: O2 100% NRB					
5. SA: Vitals					
6. TI: IV access*					
7. TI: Fluid bolus*					
8. Splint wound*					
9. Immobilize and extricate*					
10. Reassessment					
11. TI: Pain meds					
12. Transport: Emergent					
13. Reassessment					
14. TI:					
15. SA: head to toe exam					
16. Reassessment					
17. Report					
TEAMWORK/LEADERSHIP					
1. Coordination					
2. Flexibility					
3. Communication					
4. Affect: Rapport & Support					
5. Overall					

* Actions are mandatory.

SELF EVALUATION: ☐ Successful ☐ Unsuccessful

SCORE: /22

NOTES:

Potentially Harmful/Dangerous actions (omission, commission, sequencing):

C DEBRIEFING

Debriefing Questions:

1. How did you feel throughout the simulation experience?
2. What were your primary diagnoses in this scenario?
3. Did you feel you had the knowledge and skills to care for this patient? Why/ why not?
4. What were your priority assessments and interventions?
5. What outcomes did you measure?
6. What did you do well?
7. What was missed? What would you have done differently?
8. Is there anything else you would like to discuss?

Critical Thinking

1. What are your considerations if the extrication will be prolonged?

EMS PATIENT CARE REPORT (PCR) Scenario:

PATIENT INFORMATION

Name:	Allergies:
Age:	Medications:
Sex:	Past Medical History:
Weight: Kg (lb)	Chief Complaint:

VITAL SIGNS

Time:	BP:	Pulse:	Respiration:	Sao_2:
Time:	BP:	Pulse:	Respiration:	Sao_2:
Time:	BP:	Pulse:	Respiration:	Sao_2:

PHYSICAL / NEUROLOGICAL EXAM

LOC:	Skin:	AB/GI:
Oriented:	HEENT:	Pelvis:
GCS:	Neck:	GU:
Pupils:	Chest:	Posterior :
Sensory/Motor:	Respiratory:	Extremities:
Facial Droop:	Cardiovascular:	Psychiatric:
Speech:	EKG:	GLU:

CHIEF COMPLAINT

HISTORY OF PRESENT ILLNESS

NOTES

EMS PATIENT CARE REPORT (PCR) Scenario:

PATIENT INFORMATION

Name:
Age:
Sex:
Weight: Kg (lb)

Allergies:
Medications:
Past Medical History:
Chief Complaint:

VITAL SIGNS

Time:	BP:	Pulse:	Respiration:	Sao_2:
Time:	BP:	Pulse:	Respiration:	Sao_2:
Time:	BP:	Pulse:	Respiration:	Sao_2:

PHYSICAL / NEUROLOGICAL EXAM

LOC:	Skin:	AB/GI:
Oriented:	HEENT:	Pelvis:
GCS:	Neck:	GU:
Pupils:	Chest:	Posterior :
Sensory/Motor:	Respiratory:	Extremities:
Facial Droop:	Cardiovascular:	Psychiatric:
Speech:	EKG:	GLU:

CHIEF COMPLAINT

HISTORY OF PRESENT ILLNESS

NOTES

ADULT TRAUMA PENETRATING

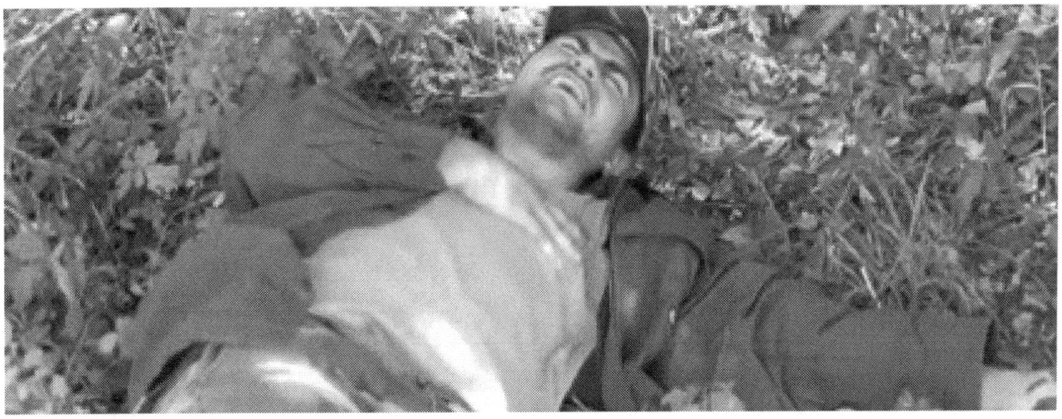

18 Y/O MALE, PENETRATING GSW TO CHEST

DISPATCH
Location: Rural road
Type of situation:Penetrating trauma
Number of patients: 1
Hazards: Unknown

OBJECTIVES

A. Assessment of the critically injured patient
B. Understand pathophysiology of tension pneumothorax
C. Recognize need for rapid transport to a trauma center
D. Recognize and treat tension pneumothorax
E. Recognition and treatment of hypovolemic shock
F. Use of long spine board for immobilization/evacuation

SCENE SIZE-UP	
OVERALL SAFETY	SCENE SAFETY UNKNOWN
MOI / NOI	PENETRATING GSW TO CHEST
RESOURCES	ALS RESPONSE
C-SPINE	SIGNS OF TRAUMA

PATHOPHYSIOLOGY

Overview:

A traumatic pneumothorax may result from both blunt trauma and penetrating injuries to the chest wall. The most common mechanism is a cut to the pleura by a fractured rib. Tension pneumothorax occurs because the opening that allows air to enter the pleural space functions like a valve, and with every breath more air enters and cannot escape. Severe hypoxia follows, with a resultant drop in blood pressure and level of consciousness.

Signs and symptoms of a tension Pnuemo is severe respiratory distress, low blood pressure, JVD, absent lung sounds on the affected side, muffled heart sounds, subcutaneous emphasema, and a late sign of tracheal deviation. Pupils in any fight or flight situation will be dilated from a sympathetic nervous system response.

A tension pneumo is treated with needle chest decompression at either the 2nd intercostals space over the top of the third rib midclavicular, or the 5th intercostals space mid axillary. Due to the potential underlying injuries with no exit wound spinal precautions are

necessary.

T3 SIMULATION SYSTEM

Penetrating Trauma GSW: Performance

Performance Checklist Role: | Start Time: End Time:

Expected Actions	Time	2	1	0	N/A
1. SSU: Spinal Immoblilzation *					
2. PS: ABCDE, full head to toe and exit wound check					
3. BVM *					
4. Occlusive dressing *					
5. Immobilize and Extricate*					
6. Transport: Emergent					
7. Reassessment					
8. SA: Vitals					
9. D DX: tension pneumotho-rax *					
10. Perform NCD *					
11. IV access and fluids *					
12 Reassessment					
13. Report					
TEAMWORK/LEADERSHIP					
1. Coordination					
2. Flexibility					
3. Communication					
4. Affect: Rapport & Support *					
5. Overall					

(*) actions are mandatory

SELF EVALUATION: ☐ Successful ☐ Unsuccessful | **SCORE:** /36

NOTES:

Potentially Harmful/ Dangerous Actions (omission, commission, sequencing):

C DEBRIEFING

Debriefing Questions:

1. What happened?
2. How did you feel throughout the simulation experience?
3. What were your priority assessments and interventions?
4. What did you do well?
5. What was missed? What would you have done differently?
6. What additional information would you need?
7. Is there anything else you would like to discuss?

Critical Thinking

1. What are the signs and symptoms of a pneumothorax?
2. What is the target range for maintaining blood pressure?

Penetrating Trauma GSW: Performance

Performance Checklist	Role:	Start Time:	End Time:

Expected Actions	Time	2	1	0	N/A
1. SSU: Spinal Immoblilzation *					
2. PS: ABCDE, full head to toe and exit wound check					
3. BVM *					
4. Attempt intubation *					
5. Surgical Airway*					
6. Immobilize and Extricate*					
7. Transport Emergent*					
8. Reassessment					
9. SA: Vitals					
10. TI: IV access and fluids *					
11. Reassessment					
12. Report					
TEAMWORK/LEADERSHIP					
1. Coordination					
2. Flexibility					
3. Communication					
4. Affect: Rapport & Support *					
5. Overall					

(*) actions are mandatory

SELF EVALUATION: ☐ **Successful** ☐ **Unsuccessful**

SCORE: /34

NOTES:

Potentially Harmful/ Dangerous Actions (omission, commission, sequencing):

C DEBRIEFING

Debriefing Questions:

1. What happened?
2. How did you feel throughout the simulation experience?
3. What were your priority assessments and interventions?
4. What did you do well?
5. What was missed? What would you have done differently?
6. What additional information would you need?
7. Is there anything else you would like to discuss?

Critical Thinking

1. What are the indications for a surgical airway?

EMS PATIENT CARE REPORT (PCR) Scenario:

PATIENT INFORMATION

Name:	Allergies:
Age:	Medications:
Sex:	Past Medical History:
Weight: Kg (lb)	Chief Complaint:

VITAL SIGNS

Time:	BP:	Pulse:	Respiration:	Sao_2:
Time:	BP:	Pulse:	Respiration:	Sao_2:
Time:	BP:	Pulse:	Respiration:	Sao_2:

PHYSICAL / NEUROLOGICAL EXAM

LOC:	Skin:	AB/GI:
Oriented:	HEENT:	Pelvis:
GCS:	Neck:	GU:
Pupils:	Chest:	Posterior :
Sensory/Motor:	Respiratory:	Extremities:
Facial Droop:	Cardiovascular:	Psychiatric:
Speech:	EKG:	GLU:

CHIEF COMPLAINT

HISTORY OF PRESENT ILLNESS

NOTES

EMS PATIENT CARE REPORT (PCR) Scenario:

PATIENT INFORMATION

Name: Age: Sex: Weight: Kg (lb)	Allergies: Medications: Past Medical History: Chief Complaint:

VITAL SIGNS

Time:	BP:	Pulse:	Respiration:	Sao_2:
Time:	BP:	Pulse:	Respiration:	Sao_2:
Time:	BP:	Pulse:	Respiration:	Sao_2:

PHYSICAL / NEUROLOGICAL EXAM

LOC: Oriented: GCS: Pupils: Sensory/Motor: Facial Droop: Speech:	Skin: HEENT: Neck: Chest: Respiratory: Cardiovascular: EKG:	AB/GI: Pelvis: GU: Posterior : Extremities: Psychiatric: GLU:

CHIEF COMPLAINT

HISTORY OF PRESENT ILLNESS

NOTES

GERIATRIC ABDOMINAL PAIN

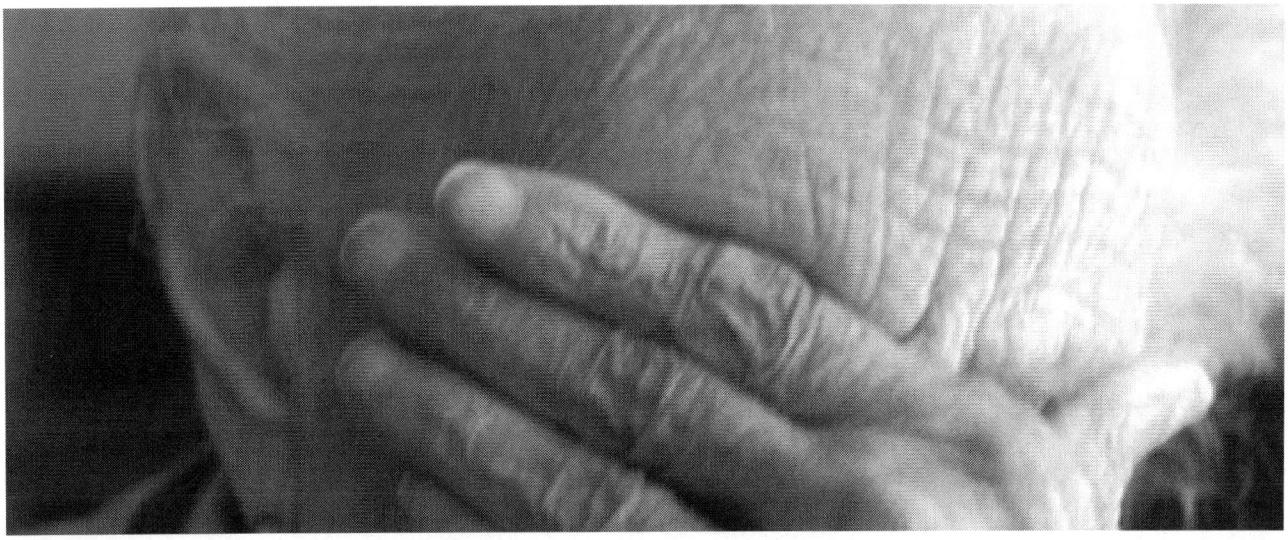

80 Y/O FEMALE, ABDOMINAL PAIN AND WEAKNESS

DISPATCH
Location: Suburban home
Type of situation: Pain and weakness
Number of patients: 1
Hazards: No hazards

OBJECTIVES

a. Assessment of the patient
b. Understanding of the pathophysiology of abdominal pain
c. Prioritization of interventions
d. Recognition of the signs and symptoms of lower bleeding and hypovolemia.
e. Performance of appropriate interventions
f. Demonstration of effective teamwork.

SCENE SIZE-UP	
OVERALL SAFETY	SCENE IS SAFE
MOI / NOI	ABDOMINAL PAIN AND WEAKNESS
RESOURCES	ALS RESPONSE
C-SPINE	NO SIGNS OF TRAUMA

PATHOPHYSIOLOGY

Overview:

Lower GI bleeds present with black, tarry, foul smelling stools. Black, tarry, blood (melena) has been in the colon for several hours, bright red blood indicates a source near the anus or vigorous bleeding in the colon.

Lower GI bleeding is most commonly from diverticulitis an infection in an out-pouching of the large intestine. Fecal material will collect in this pouch and irritate the mucosa. Diverticulitis can bleed aggressively. Other sources of melena are from upper GI bleed or colon cancer. It takes approximately 200 cc of blood in the large bowel to create melena. Treatment should be supportive. Assessment for hypotension can be based on vitals or a tilt test. If the patient presents with significant hypotension then aggressive fluid resuscitation may have to be implemented. Up to 2 liters of NaCl can be infused before blood products should be given. Since most patients with lower GI bleeding are elderly and have comorbid medical conditions, fluid resuscitation should be done carefully.

GI Bleed: Performance

Performance Checklist | Role: | Start Time: | End Time:

Expected Actions	Time	2	1	0	N/A
1. Scene Size-up: Safety *					
2. Primary Survey: CC, LOC, HPI					
3. Primary Survey: ABCs					
4. SA: Vitals					
5. TI: Lay supine *					
6. TI: 100% O2 by NC					
7. SA: Abdominal Inspection					
8. SA: 12 lead EKG *					
9. SA: Blood sugar *					
10. Diff Diagnosis: GI Bleed *					
11. Transport: Non-Emergent					
12. Reassessment					
13. TI: IV Access & Fluids *					
14. TI: 2nd line					
15. Reassessment					
16. Report					
TEAMWORK/LEADERSHIP					
1. Coordination					
2. Flexibility					
3. Communication					
4. Affect: Rapport & Support					
5. Overall					

(*) Actions are mandatory

SELF EVALUATION: ☐ Successful ☐ Unsuccessful

SCORE: /42

NOTES:

Potentially Harmful/Dangerous actions (omission, commission, sequencing) :

C DEBRIEFING

Debriefing Questions:

1. How did you feel throughout the simulation experience?
2. What were your primary diagnoses in this scenario?
3. Did you feel you had the knowledge and skills to care for this patient? Why/ why not?
4. What were your priority assessments and interventions?
5. What outcomes did you measure?
6. What did you do well?
7. What was missed? What would you have done differently?
8. Is there anything else you would like to discuss?

Critical Thinking

1. What is major cause of lower GI bleeding in the elderly?

2. What does the black tarry stool contain?

3. What is the most likely source of bright red blood from the rectum?

Abdominal Pain

Performance Checklist | Role: | Start Time: | End Time:

Expected Actions	Time	2	1	0	N/A
1. Scene Size-up: Safety *					
2. Primary Survey: CC, LOC, HPI					
3. Primary Survey: ABCs					
4. SA: Vitals					
5. TI: Lay supine *					
6. TI: 100% O2 by NC					
7. SA: Abdominal Inspection					
8. SA: 12 lead EKG *					
9. SA: Blood sugar *					
10. Diff Diagnosis:					
11. Transport: Emergent					
12. Reassessment					
13. TI: IV Access & Fluids *					
14. TI: 2nd line					
15. Reassessment					
16. Report					
TEAMWORK/LEADERSHIP					
1. Coordination					
2. Flexibility					
3. Communication					
4. Affect: Rapport & Support					
5. Overall					

(*) Actions are mandatory

SELF EVALUATION: ☐ Successful ☐ Unsuccessful | **SCORE: /42**

NOTES:

Potentially Harmful/Dangerous actions (omission, commission, sequencing) :

C DEBRIEFING

Debriefing Questions:

1. How did you feel throughout the simulation experience?
2. What were your primary diagnoses in this scenario?
3. Did you feel you had the knowledge and skills to care for this patient? Why/ why not?
4. What were your priority assessments and interventions?
5. What outcomes did you measure?
6. What did you do well?
7. What was missed? What would you have done differently?
8. Is there anything else you would like to discuss?

Critical Thinking

1- How would you distinguish between upper and lower GI bleed?

2- What are some of the most common causes of upper GI bleed?

EMS PATIENT CARE REPORT (PCR) Scenario:

PATIENT INFORMATION

Name:	Allergies:
Age:	Medications:
Sex:	Past Medical History:
Weight: Kg (lb)	Chief Complaint:

VITAL SIGNS

Time:	BP:	Pulse:	Respiration:	Sao_2:
Time:	BP:	Pulse:	Respiration:	Sao_2:
Time:	BP:	Pulse:	Respiration:	Sao_2:

PHYSICAL / NEUROLOGICAL EXAM

LOC:	Skin:	AB/GI:
Oriented:	HEENT:	Pelvis:
GCS:	Neck:	GU:
Pupils:	Chest:	Posterior :
Sensory/Motor:	Respiratory:	Extremities:
Facial Droop:	Cardiovascular:	Psychiatric:
Speech:	EKG:	GLU:

CHIEF COMPLAINT

HISTORY OF PRESENT ILLNESS

NOTES

EMS PATIENT CARE REPORT (PCR) Scenario:

PATIENT INFORMATION

Name:	Allergies:
Age:	Medications:
Sex:	Past Medical History:
Weight: Kg (lb)	Chief Complaint:

VITAL SIGNS

Time:	BP:	Pulse:	Respiration:	Sao_2:
Time:	BP:	Pulse:	Respiration:	Sao_2:
Time:	BP:	Pulse:	Respiration:	Sao_2:

PHYSICAL / NEUROLOGICAL EXAM

LOC:	Skin:	AB/GI:
Oriented:	HEENT:	Pelvis:
GCS:	Neck:	GU:
Pupils:	Chest:	Posterior :
Sensory/Motor:	Respiratory:	Extremities:
Facial Droop:	Cardiovascular:	Psychiatric:
Speech:	EKG:	GLU:

CHIEF COMPLAINT

HISTORY OF PRESENT ILLNESS

NOTES

GERIATRIC CARDIAC RHYTHM DISTURBANCE

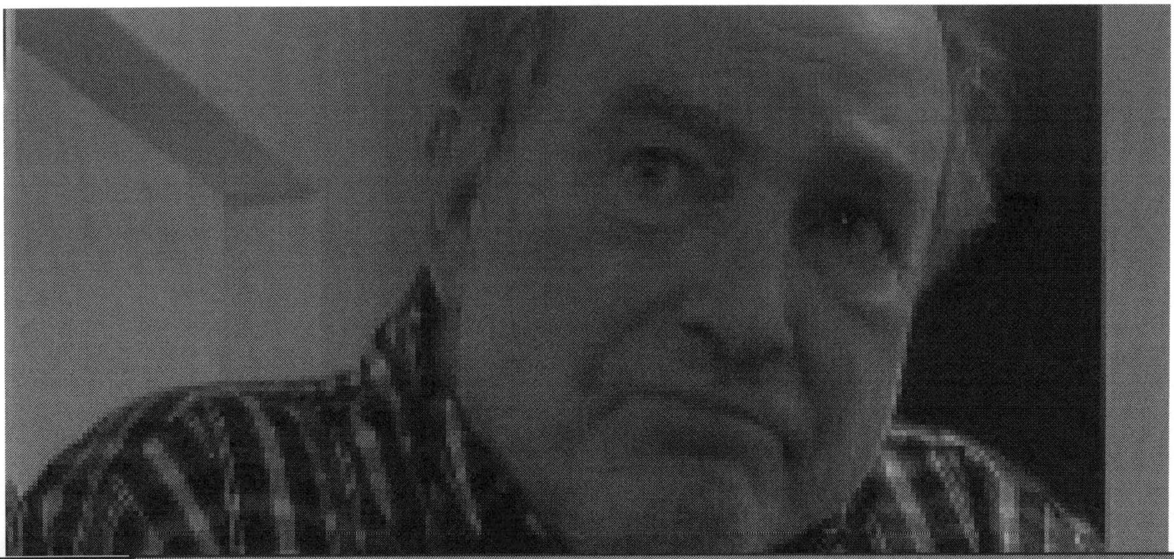

80 Y/O MALE, CHEST PAIN AND WEAKNESS

DISPATCH
Location: Apartment
Type of situation: Chest pain and weakness
Number of patients: 1
Hazards: No hazards

OBJECTIVES

1. Assessment of the scene and the patient.
2. Recognition of the signs and symptoms of cardiac compromise
3. Understand the pathophysiology of the cardiovascular system.
4. Explain the principles of CPR, AED use and resuscitation
5. Prioritization of interventions and treatment.
6. Teamwork, communication and division of duties

SCENE SIZE-UP	
OVERALL SAFETY	SCENE IS SAFE
MOI / NOI	CHEST PAIN AND WEAKNESS
RESOURCES	BLS RESPONSE
C-SPINE	NO SIGNS OF TRAUMA

PATHOPHYSIOLOGY

Overview:

Bradycardia is defined as a heart rate under than 60, or under 50 if on a beta blocker drug. There are multiple causes of bradycardia including medications, poisoning, increased vagal tone, and cardiac conduction abnormalities. Syncope or near syncope while sitting down should be assumed to be cardiac until proven otherwise.

Treatment will be based upon signs or symptoms of poor perfusion, and the type of bradycardia. If the patient is in a type II second degree or a 3rd degree block with chest pain, dyspnea, decreased LOC, hypotension, shock , pulmonary edema or having a MI, transcutaneous pacing should immediately begin. Sedation should be used as needed and if blood pressure allows.

If the patient has stable symptoms and is bradycardic, and the bradycardia is not from Mobitz type II or 3rd degree, an atropine trial can be administered.

Atropine will probably not be effective for blocks that are below the AV node. (Mobitz type II and 3rd degree). Atropine and pacing may not work for certain types of overdoses. (Calcium Channel)

Cardiac Bradycardia: Performance

Performance Checklist

Role:	Start Time:	End Time:

Expected Actions	Time	2	1	0	N/A
1.Scene Size-up*					
2. PS : CC, LOC, HPI					
3. PS: ABCs					
4. TI: 100% 02 by NRB					
5. TI: Aspirin					
6. Secondary Assessment- Vitals, PMH					
7. SA: Blood sugar					
8. TI: Patient positioning					
9. IV access and fluids					
10. Obtain EKG*					
11. Differential DX- 3rd degree block*					
12. TI: Sedation Versed					
13. TI: Pace*					
14. Transport: Emergent to Cath Lab*					
15. Reassessment					
TEAMWORK/LEADERSHIP					
1. Coordination of Treatment					
2. Communication					
3. Situational Awareness					
4. Affect					
5. Overall					

*RED actions are Mandatory

SELF EVALUATION: ☐ Successful ☐ Unsuccessful

SCORE: /40

NOTES:

Potentially Harmful/ Dangerous Actions (omission, commission, sequencing):

C DEBRIEFING

Debriefing Questions:

1. How did feel throughout the simulation experience?
2. What were your primary diagnoses in this scenario?
3. Did you feel you had the knowledge and skills to care for this patient? Why/ why not?
4. What were your priority assessments and interventions?
5. What outcomes did you measure?
6. What did you do well?
7. What was missed? What would you have done differently?
8. Is there anything else you would like to discuss?

Critical Thinking:

1. What is the greatest priority with this call?
2. What is the best way to achieve this?
3. Why not give atropine first?
4. What may happen if we don't get the appropriate treatment going right away?

T3 SIMULATION SYSTEM

Cardiac Performance

Performance Checklist

Role:	Start Time:	End Time:

Expected Actions	Time	2	1	0	N/A
1.Scene Size-up*					
2. PS : CC, LOC, HPI					
3. PS: ABCs					
4. TI: 100% 02 by NRB					
5. TI:					
6. Secondary Assessment-Vitals, PMH					
7. SA: Blood sugar					
8. TI:					
9. IV access and fluids					
10. Obtain EKG*					
11. Differential DX*					
12. TI: Atropine*					
13. TI:					
14. Transport:					
15. Reassessment					
16.TI:					
17. Report					
TEAMWORK/LEADERSHIP					
1. Coordination of Treatment					
2. Communication					
3. Situational Awareness					
4. Affect					
5. Overall					

*RED actions are Mandatory

SELF EVALUATION: ☐ Successful ☐ Unsuccessful

SCORE: /44

NOTES:

Potentially Harmful/ Dangerous Actions (omission, commission, sequencing):

C DEBRIEFING

Debriefing Questions:

1. How did feel throughout the simulation experience?
2. What were your primary diagnoses in this scenario?
3. Did you feel you had the knowledge and skills to care for this patient? Why/ why not?
4. What were your priority assessments and interventions?
5. What outcomes did you measure?
6. What did you do well?
7. What was missed? What would you have done differently?
8. Is there anything else you would like to discuss?

Critical Thinking:

1. What is the greatest priority with this call?

2. How do you determine if the patient is stable or unstable?

EMS PATIENT CARE REPORT (PCR) Scenario:

PATIENT INFORMATION

Name:	Allergies:
Age:	Medications:
Sex:	Past Medical History:
Weight: Kg (lb)	Chief Complaint:

VITAL SIGNS

Time:	BP:	Pulse:	Respiration:	Sao_2:
Time:	BP:	Pulse:	Respiration:	Sao_2:
Time:	BP:	Pulse:	Respiration:	Sao_2:

PHYSICAL / NEUROLOGICAL EXAM

LOC:	Skin:	AB/GI:
Oriented:	HEENT:	Pelvis:
GCS:	Neck:	GU:
Pupils:	Chest:	Posterior :
Sensory/Motor:	Respiratory:	Extremities:
Facial Droop:	Cardiovascular:	Psychiatric:
Speech:	EKG:	GLU:

CHIEF COMPLAINT

HISTORY OF PRESENT ILLNESS

NOTES

EMS PATIENT CARE REPORT (PCR) Scenario:

PATIENT INFORMATION

Name:	Allergies:
Age:	Medications:
Sex:	Past Medical History:
Weight: Kg (lb)	Chief Complaint:

VITAL SIGNS

Time:	BP:	Pulse:	Respiration:	Sao_2:
Time:	BP:	Pulse:	Respiration:	Sao_2:
Time:	BP:	Pulse:	Respiration:	Sao_2:

PHYSICAL / NEUROLOGICAL EXAM

LOC:	Skin:	AB/GI:
Oriented:	HEENT:	Pelvis:
GCS:	Neck:	GU:
Pupils:	Chest:	Posterior :
Sensory/Motor:	Respiratory:	Extremities:
Facial Droop:	Cardiovascular:	Psychiatric:
Speech:	EKG:	GLU:

CHIEF COMPLAINT

HISTORY OF PRESENT ILLNESS

NOTES

GERIATRIC RESPIRATORY

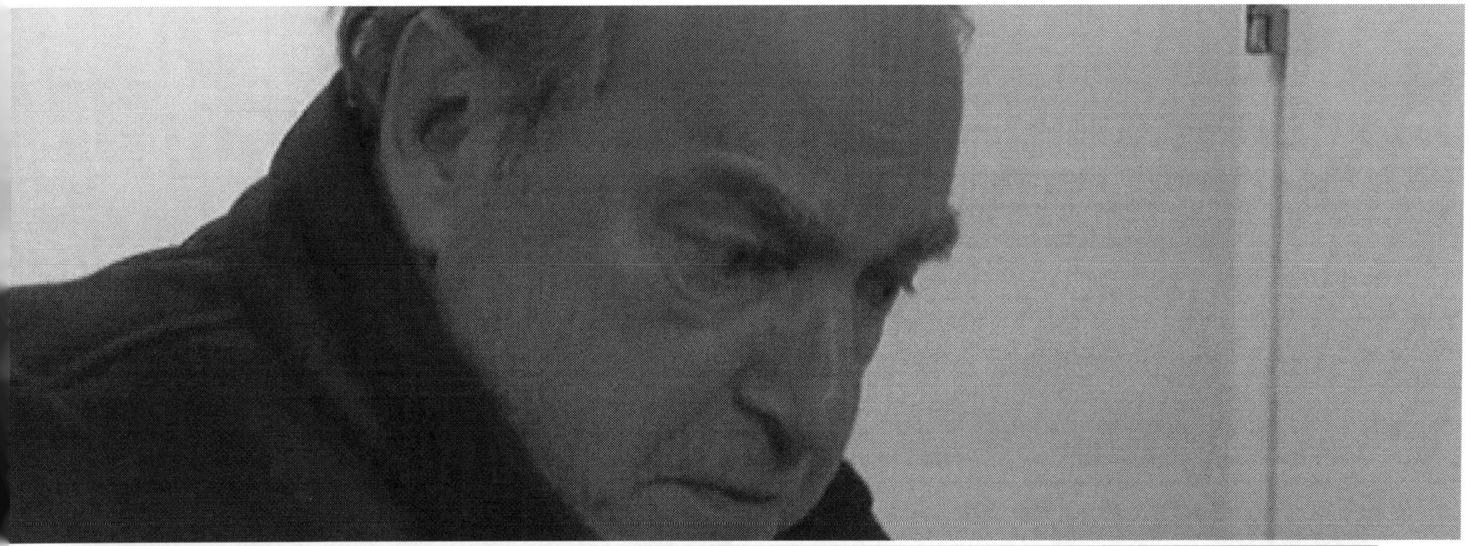

68 Y/O MALE, SHORTNESS OF BREATH

DISPATCH
Location: Suburban home
Type of situation:SOB, difficulty breathing
Number of patients: 1
Hazards: No hazards

OBJECTIVES
1. Assessment of the COPD patient
2. Understand the pathophysiology of COPD
3. Recognition of exacerbation of COPD
4. Prioritization and performance of interventions- O2, Nebulizer, CPAP
5. Recognition of exacerbation of COPD

SCENE SIZE-UP	
OVERALL SAFETY	SCENE IS SAFE
MOI / NOI	SHORTNESS OF BREATH
RESOURCES	ALS RESPONSE
C-SPINE	NO SIGNS OF TRAUMA

PATHOPHYSIOLOGY

Overview:

Chronic Obstructive Pulmonary Disease (COPD) is a group of pulmonary disorders that result in abnormal ventilation. The three most common diseases of COPD are: Emphysema- the destruction of the terminal alveoli, Chronic Bronchitis- increased mucus production in the entire respiratory system including the alveoli, and Asthma-a chronic inflammatory disorder of the airways that includes bronchoconstriction, and excessive mucus production. The result is significant air trapping in the distal bronchioles and alveoli. This results in an increase in CO_2, a decrease in O_2 and difficulty in exhaling. COPD is a chronic disease that can become much worse with an infection like pneumonia or bronchitis. The most common cause of COPD is smoking.

While chronic COPD is not reversible, acute episodes can be treated. Treatment is increased oxygen administration, reversal of the bronchospasm with a beta-adrenergic agent- albuterol,or levabuterol (Xopenex), diminishing mucus production - ipratropium (Atrovent), and preventing the inflammatory response- corticosteroids.

Patient position is also very important, the patient should be allowed to sit upright as possible, and encouraged to purse lip breathe. Oxygen therapy should be given to maintain a $SaO_2 > 95$ %.

The goal is to reduce the air trapping and CO_2 level; low oxygen saturation is a late and serious sign in COPD.

Respiratory Distress COPD: Performance

Performance Checklist | Role: | Start Time: End Time:

Expected Actions	Time	2	1	0	N/A
1. Scene Size-up :Address Safety*					
2. PS: CC, LOC, HPI					
3. PS: ABC					
4. TI: 100% 02					
5. SA: Vital Signs, History					
6. DD: COPD Exacerbation*					
7. TI: Nebulizer Treatment*					
8. Transport: Non-emergent*					
9. Reassessment: ABC, Vitals					
10. Place Patient on Monitor					
11. TI: CPAP*					
12. TI: IV Access*					
13. 12 Lead EKG*					
14. Transparent Thinking					
15. Medication Solumedrol					
16. Communication: Med Control					
17. TI: Intervention 2nd Nebulizer*					
18. Report					
TEAMWORK/LEADERSHIP					
1. Coordination					
2. Flexibility					
3. Communication					
4. Affect: Rapport & Support*					
5. Overall					

SELF EVALUATION: ☐ Successful ☐ Unsuccessful

SCORE: /46

NOTES:

Potentially harmful/dangerous actions (omission, commission, sequencing):

C DEBRIEFING

Debriefing Questions:

1. How did feel throughout the simulation experience?
2. What were your priority assessments and interventions? What concerns did you have about this patient?
3. What was significant about the client's history? Did you notice low SP02 in a timely fashion and increased anxiety?
4. What did you do well?
5. What was missed? What would you have done differently?
6. What are the important teaching points for this patient and his family
7. Is there anything else you would like to discuss?

Critical Thinking

1. What is the most serious concern for this patient?
2. What is the cause of most exacerbations of COPD?
3. What additional treatment can a medic provide ?
4. What is the best technique to bag a COPD patient who is tight?

Respiratory Failure COPD: Performance

Performance	Role:	Start Time:	End Time:

Expected Actions	Time	2	1	0	N/A
1. Scene Size-up :Address Safety*					
2. PS: CC, LOC, HPI					
3. PS: ABC					
4. TI: 100% 02					
5. SA: Vital Signs, History					
6. DD: COPD Exacerbation*					
7. TI: Nebulizer Treatment*					
8. Transport: Non-emergent*					
9. Reassessment: ABC, Vitals					
10. Place Patient on Monitor					
11. TI: CPAP*					
12. TI: IV Access*					
13. 12 Lead EKG*					
14. Transparent Thinking					
15. TI: Intubation*					
16. Communication: Med Control					
17. TI:					
18. Report					
TEAMWORK/LEADERSHIP					
1. Coordination					
2. Flexibility					
3. Communication					
4. Affect: Rapport & Support*					
5. Overall					

SELF EVALUATION: ☐ Successful ☐ Unsuccessful

SCORE: /46

NOTES:

Potentially harmful/dangerous actions (omission, commission, sequencing):

C DEBRIEFING

Debriefing Questions:

1. How did feel throughout the simulation experience?
2. What were your priority assessments and interventions? What concerns did you have about this patient?
3. What was significant about the client's history? Did you notice low SP02 in a timely fashion and increased anxiety?
4. What did you do well?
5. What was missed? What would you have done differently?
6. What are the important teaching points for this patient and his family
7. Is there anything else you would like to discuss?

Critical Thinking

1. Why do these patients go into respiratory failure?

EMS PATIENT CARE REPORT (PCR) Scenario:

PATIENT INFORMATION

Name:	Allergies:
Age:	Medications:
Sex:	Past Medical History:
Weight: Kg (lb)	Chief Complaint:

VITAL SIGNS

Time:	BP:	Pulse:	Respiration:	Sao_2:
Time:	BP:	Pulse:	Respiration:	Sao_2:
Time:	BP:	Pulse:	Respiration:	Sao_2:

PHYSICAL / NEUROLOGICAL EXAM

LOC:	Skin:	AB/GI:
Oriented:	HEENT:	Pelvis:
GCS:	Neck:	GU:
Pupils:	Chest:	Posterior :
Sensory/Motor:	Respiratory:	Extremities:
Facial Droop:	Cardiovascular:	Psychiatric:
Speech:	EKG:	GLU:

CHIEF COMPLAINT

HISTORY OF PRESENT ILLNESS

NOTES

EMS PATIENT CARE REPORT (PCR) Scenario:

PATIENT INFORMATION

Name:	Allergies:
Age:	Medications:
Sex:	Past Medical History:
Weight: Kg (lb)	Chief Complaint:

VITAL SIGNS

Time:	BP:	Pulse:	Respiration:	Sao_2:
Time:	BP:	Pulse:	Respiration:	Sao_2:
Time:	BP:	Pulse:	Respiration:	Sao_2:

PHYSICAL / NEUROLOGICAL EXAM

LOC:	Skin:	AB/GI:
Oriented:	HEENT:	Pelvis:
GCS:	Neck:	GU:
Pupils:	Chest:	Posterior :
Sensory/Motor:	Respiratory:	Extremities:
Facial Droop:	Cardiovascular:	Psychiatric:
Speech:	EKG:	GLU:

CHIEF COMPLAINT

HISTORY OF PRESENT ILLNESS

NOTES

GERIATRIC SEPSIS

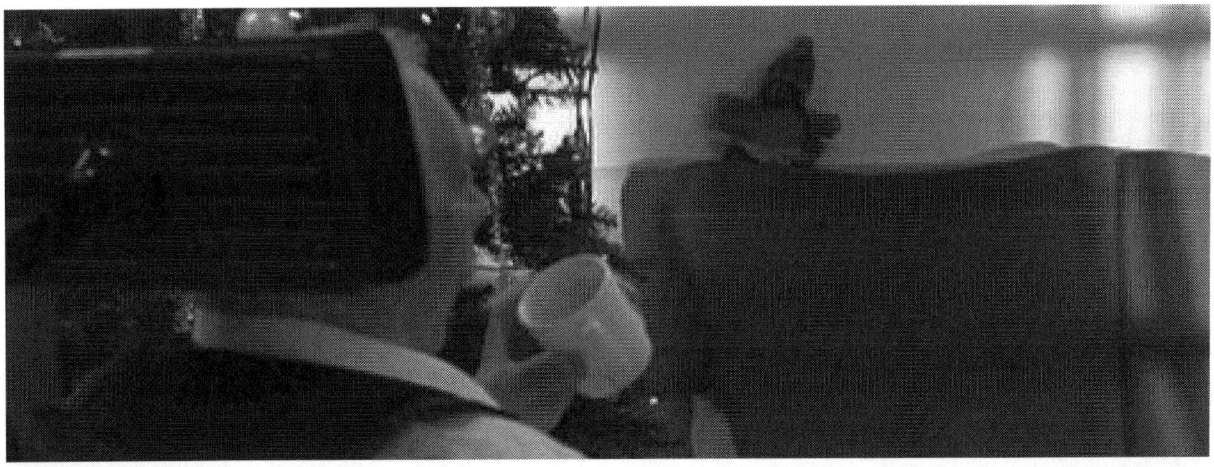

85 Y/O MALE
ALTERED MENTAL STATUS

DISPATCH
Location: Nursing home
Type of situation: AMS
Time of Day: 08:30 pm
Number of patients: 1
Hazards: Scene is safe

OBJECTIVES

1. Understand the pathophysiology of sepsis.
2. Recognition signs and symptoms of uro-sepsis
3. Identify sepsis in a venerable population
4. Prioritize interventions.
5. Perform appropriate interventions

SCENE SIZE-UP	
OVERALL SAFETY	SCENE IS SAFE
MOI / NOI	CHANGE
RESOURCES	ALS RESPONSE
C-SPINE	NO SIGNS OF TRAUMA

PATHOPHYSIOLOGY

Overview:

An elderly patient (especially a female) with an unexplained fever, decrease in LOC and an indwelling urinary catheter should be highly suspicious of uro-sepsis. Sepsis is a pre-hospital emergency and needs to be immediately treated with aggressive fluid resuscitation.

Sepsis is the whole body inflammatory response to waste products of a bacterial infection.
The original site of infection can be anywhere, the GU (UTI, kidney infection), GI (peritonitis, pancreatitis, gall bladder, and liver), Respiratory (pneumonia), Skin (cellulitis, burns). The infection travels from the original site into the vascular system and causes other body systems to have the inflammatory response. Severe sepsis is defined as: Heart rate > 90 bpm, Temperature > 100.4 F (38C) or < 96.8 F (36C), RR> 20, Mottled skin, altered mental status, cardiac dysfunction, (low cardiac output).

Treatment: High Flow O_2, IV Fluids (MAP> 65), Dopamine (if unable to keep MAP > 65 with 2 L of NaCl.

T3 SIMULATION SYSTEM

SEPSIS

Performance Checklist Role: Start Time: End Time:

Expected Actions	Time	2	1	0	N/A
1. Scene Size-up: Safety					
2. Primary Survey: CC, LOC, HPI					
3. Primary Survey: ABCs					
4. Initial Assessment					
5. 100% O_2					
6. Airway Management					
7. IV access*					
8. Rapid fluid bolus up to 2 L of NaCl*					
9. Consider Dopamine 2-20 mcg/kg/min					
10. Rapid transport*					
11. Reassessment					
12. Report					
* Critical Actions					
TEAMWORK/LEADERSHIP					
1. Coordination					
2. Flexibility					
3. Communication					
4. Affect: Rapport & Support					
5. Overall					

SELF EVALUATION: ☐ Successful ☐ Unsuccessful

SCORE: /34

NOTES:

C DEBRIEFING

Debriefing Questions:

1. How did feel throughout the simulation experience?
2. What were your primary diagnoses in this scenario?
3. Did you feel you had the knowledge and skills to care for this patient? Why/ why not?
4. What were your priority assessments and interventions?
5. What outcomes did you measure?
6. What did you do well?
7. What was missed? What would you have done differently?
8. Is there anything else you would like to discuss?

Critical Thinking

1. How does an infection become sepsis?
2. What are some common sources of infection that become sepsis?

SEPSIS

Performance Checklist Role: | Start Time: End Time:

Expected Actions	Time	2	1	0	N/A
1. Scene Size-up: Safety					
2. Primary Survey: CC, LOC, HPI					
3. Primary Survey: ABCs					
4. Initial Assessment					
5. 100% O_2					
6. Airway Management					
7. IV access*					
8. Rapid fluid bolus up to 2 L of NaCl*					
9. Consider Dopamine 2-20 mcg/kg/min					
10. Rapid transport*					
11. Reassessment					
12. Report					
* Critical Actions					
TEAMWORK/LEADERSHIP					
1. Coordination					
2. Flexibility					
3. Communication					
4. Affect: Rapport & Support					
5. Overall					

SELF EVALUATION: ☐ Successful ☐ Unsuccessful

SCORE: /34

NOTES:

C DEBRIEFING

Debriefing Questions:

1. How did feel throughout the simulation experience?
2. What were your primary diagnoses in this scenario?
3. Did you feel you had the knowledge and skills to care for this patient? Why/ why not?
4. What were your priority assessments and interventions?
5. What outcomes did you measure?
6. What did you do well?
7. What was missed? What would you have done differently?
8. Is there anything else you would like to discuss?

Critical Thinking

1. Why is aggressive fluid resuscitation so important in sepsis?

EMS PATIENT CARE REPORT (PCR) Scenario:

PATIENT INFORMATION

Name:	Allergies:
Age:	Medications:
Sex:	Past Medical History:
Weight: Kg (lb)	Chief Complaint:

VITAL SIGNS

Time:	BP:	Pulse:	Respiration:	Sao_2:
Time:	BP:	Pulse:	Respiration:	Sao_2:
Time:	BP:	Pulse:	Respiration:	Sao_2:

PHYSICAL / NEUROLOGICAL EXAM

LOC:	Skin:	AB/GI:
Oriented:	HEENT:	Pelvis:
GCS:	Neck:	GU:
Pupils:	Chest:	Posterior :
Sensory/Motor:	Respiratory:	Extremities:
Facial Droop:	Cardiovascular:	Psychiatric:
Speech:	EKG:	GLU:

CHIEF COMPLAINT

HISTORY OF PRESENT ILLNESS

NOTES

EMS PATIENT CARE REPORT (PCR) Scenario:

PATIENT INFORMATION

Name:	Allergies:
Age:	Medications:
Sex:	Past Medical History:
Weight: Kg (lb)	Chief Complaint:

VITAL SIGNS

Time:	BP:	Pulse:	Respiration:	Sao_2:
Time:	BP:	Pulse:	Respiration:	Sao_2:
Time:	BP:	Pulse:	Respiration:	Sao_2:

PHYSICAL / NEUROLOGICAL EXAM

LOC:	Skin:	AB/GI:
Oriented:	HEENT:	Pelvis:
GCS:	Neck:	GU:
Pupils:	Chest:	Posterior :
Sensory/Motor:	Respiratory:	Extremities:
Facial Droop:	Cardiovascular:	Psychiatric:
Speech:	EKG:	GLU:

CHIEF COMPLAINT

HISTORY OF PRESENT ILLNESS

NOTES

GERIATRIC STROKE

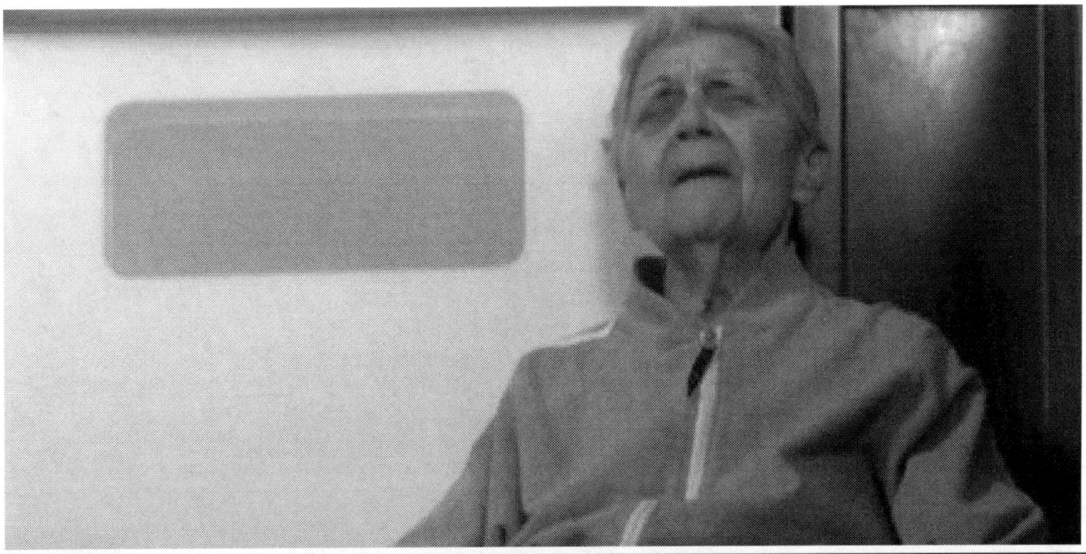

80 Y/O FEMALE, ALTERED MENTAL STATUS, POSSIBLE STROKE

DISPATCH
Location: Suburban home
Type of situation:AMS, possible stroke
Number of patients: 1
Hazards: No hazards

OBJECTIVES
1. Describe the Assessment and Treatment of a patient with a possible stroke
2. Demonstrate the use of a stroke assessment scale
3. Recognize other possible altered mental status causes
3. Prioritize and perform appropriate interventions.
5. Discuss the importance of transport destination and medical communication
6. Demonstrate effective teamwork

SCENE SIZE-UP	
OVERALL SAFETY	SCENE IS SAFE
MOI / NOI	ALTERED MENTAL STATUS, POSSIBLE STROKE
RESOURCES	ALS RESPONSE
C-SPINE	NO SIGNS OF TRAUMA

PATHOPHYSIOLOGY

Overview:

Strokes can be either a bleed or a blockage. The Blockage can be an embolus of some sort or a thrombus. Fat emboli, blood clots, plaque, or some other emboli will obstruct a vessel in the brain and cut off circulation. Ischemic stroke now have a door to drug time of up to 6 hours. TPA, (Tissue Plasminogen activator) is a clot busting drug with several contraindications. A CAT scan rules out a bleed in the brain, which would make the TPA lethal.

Stroke patients may present with some type of unilateral paralysis, facial droop, speech impediments, confusion, aphasia. Aphasia can be cognitive or expressive, in that the patient loses the ability to either express the thought in understandable words, or understand the words as spoken to them. There are different degrees of aphasia. Our role in EMS is to comfort the patient and help them find a non verbal form of communication. Blinking, Touching the hand, once for yes, twice for no. Loss of function by paralysis, with loss of communication creates significant fear and frustration. The crew must explain everything often and reassure the patient. A brain attack, or CVA can also cause swelling in the brain similar to a head injury. Unilateral pupil dilation is a sign of internal structural damage to the brain. Often stroke patients will have left or right sided gaze, which may be looking in the direction away from the affected side of the brain. Treatment is based on symptoms. Travel to the right facility is paramount, since time is a factor. Patients that have A-FIB that are non-compliant with their meds are potential stroke patients. A-Fib can cause clots to form on the ventrical walls. (Mural thrombus)

T3 SIMULATION SYSTEM

Stroke: Performance

Performance Checklist	Role:	Start Time:	End Time:

Expected Actions	Time	2	1	0	N/A
1. Scene SU: Address Safety *					
2. Primary Survey: CC. LOC, HPI					
3. Primary Survey: ABC					
4. Affect: Rapport with Pt.					
5. Assess: Blood Sugar					
6. 2nd Asses.: Neuro Exam *					
7. 2nd Asses: Vitals					
8. Therapeutic Invt: 100% O2 NC					
9. Past Medical History					
10. Diff Dx: Positive Stroke Scale *					
11. Transport:: Non-emergent to Stroke Center *					
12. Reassessment: ABC, Vitals, Neurological					
13. Comm: Early Notification *					
14, Therapeutic Int.: IV Access					
15. 12-Lead EKG					
16. Report					
TEAMWORK/LEADERSHIP					
1. Coordination					
2. Flexibility					
3. Communication					
4. Affect: Rapport & Support					
5. Overall					

(*) actions are mandatory

SELF EVALUATION: ☐ Successful ☐ Unsuccessful	SCORE: /42

NOTES:

Potentially Harmful/ Dangerous Actions (omission, commission, sequencing):

C DEBRIEFING

Debriefing Questions:

1. What happened?
2. How did you feel throughout the simulation experience?
3. What were your priority assessments and interventions?
4. What did you do well?
5. What was missed? What would you have done differently?
6. What additional information would you need?
7. Is there anything else you would like to discuss?

Critical Thinking

1. What past medical history information is relevant for stroke patients?
2. What are the transport considerations for a stroke patient?

Stroke: Performance

Performance Checklist	Role:	Start Time:	End Time:

Expected Actions	Time	2	1	0	N/A
1. Scene SU: Address Safety *					
2. Primary Survey: CC. LOC, HPI					
3. Primary Survey: ABC					
4. Affect: Rapport with Pt.					
5. Assess: Blood Sugar					
6. 2nd Asses.: Neuro Exam *					
7. 2nd Asses: Vitals					
8. Therapeutic Invt: 100% O2 NC					
9. Past Medical History					
10. Diff Dx: Positive Stroke Scale *					
11. Transport:: Non-emergent to Stroke Center *					
12. Reassessment: ABC, Vitals, Neurological					
13. Comm: Early Notification *					
14, Therapeutic Int.: IV Access					
15. 12-Lead EKG					
16. Report					
TEAMWORK/LEADERSHIP					
1. Coordination					
2. Flexibility					
3. Communication					
4. Affect: Rapport & Support					
5. Overall					

(*) actions are mandatory

SELF EVALUATION: ☐ **Successful** ☐ **Unsuccessful**

SCORE: /42

NOTES:

Potentially Harmful/ Dangerous Actions (omission, commission, sequencing):

C DEBRIEFING

Debriefing Questions:

1. What happened?
2. How did you feel throughout the simulation experience?
3. What were your priority assessments and interventions?
4. What did you do well?
5. What was missed? What would you have done differently?
6. What additional information would you need?
7. Is there anything else you would like to discuss?

Critical Thinking

1. Distinguish between a hemorrhagic stroke and an ischemic stroke.

EMS PATIENT CARE REPORT (PCR) Scenario:

PATIENT INFORMATION

Name:	Allergies:
Age:	Medications:
Sex:	Past Medical History:
Weight: Kg (lb)	Chief Complaint:

VITAL SIGNS

Time:	BP:	Pulse:	Respiration:	Sao_2:
Time:	BP:	Pulse:	Respiration:	Sao_2:
Time:	BP:	Pulse:	Respiration:	Sao_2:

PHYSICAL / NEUROLOGICAL EXAM

LOC:	Skin:	AB/GI:
Oriented:	HEENT:	Pelvis:
GCS:	Neck:	GU:
Pupils:	Chest:	Posterior :
Sensory/Motor:	Respiratory:	Extremities:
Facial Droop:	Cardiovascular:	Psychiatric:
Speech:	EKG:	GLU:

CHIEF COMPLAINT

HISTORY OF PRESENT ILLNESS

NOTES

EMS PATIENT CARE REPORT (PCR) Scenario:

PATIENT INFORMATION

Name:	Allergies:
Age:	Medications:
Sex:	Past Medical History:
Weight: Kg (lb)	Chief Complaint:

VITAL SIGNS

Time:	BP:	Pulse:	Respiration:	Sao_2:
Time:	BP:	Pulse:	Respiration:	Sao_2:
Time:	BP:	Pulse:	Respiration:	Sao_2:

PHYSICAL / NEUROLOGICAL EXAM

LOC:	Skin:	AB/GI:
Oriented:	HEENT:	Pelvis:
GCS:	Neck:	GU:
Pupils:	Chest:	Posterior :
Sensory/Motor:	Respiratory:	Extremities:
Facial Droop:	Cardiovascular:	Psychiatric:
Speech:	EKG:	GLU:

CHIEF COMPLAINT

HISTORY OF PRESENT ILLNESS

NOTES

OB-GYN DELIVERY

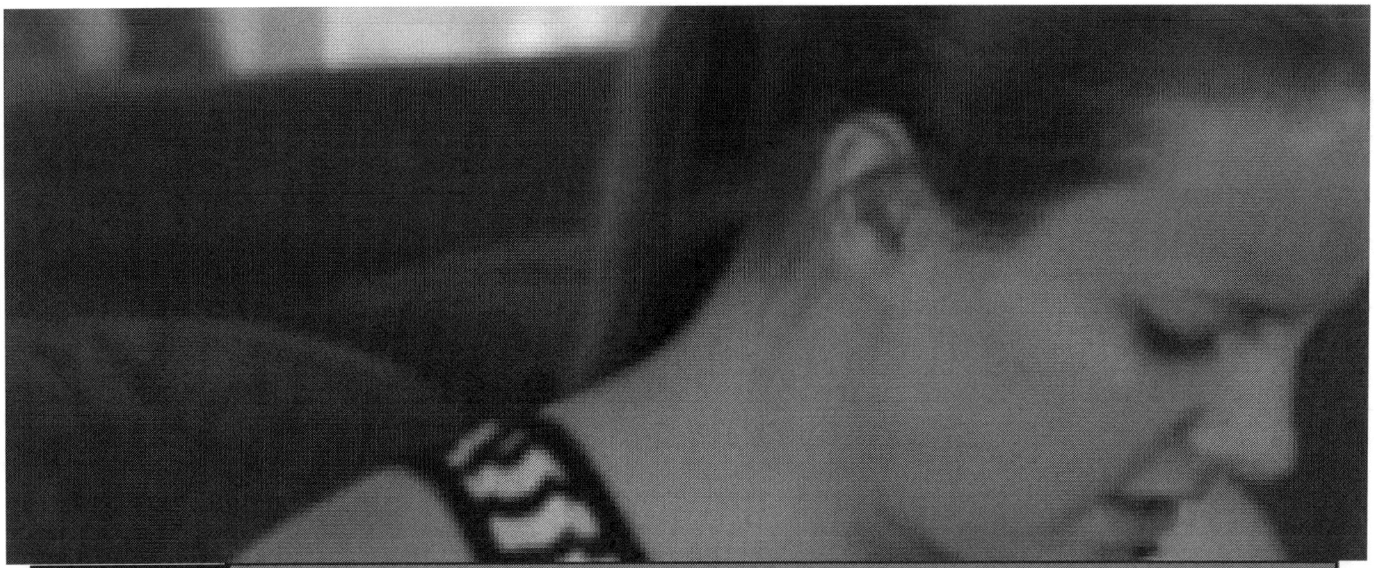

24 Y/O FEMALE, IMMINENT BIRTH

DISPATCH

Location: Suburban home
Type of situation: 38 weeks pregnant, water broke, contractions
Number of patients: 2
Hazards: No hazards

OBJECTIVES

1. Assessment of the mother before, during and after birth
2. Recognize imminent birth
3. Assessment of the newborn
4. Understanding of the pathophysiology of birth
5. Prioritization of interventions for uncomplicated delivery of term newborn and placenta
6. Recognize complicated birth situations and appropriate responses
7. Demonstration of effective teamwork

SCENE SIZE-UP	
OVERALL SAFETY	SCENE IS SAFE
MOI / NOI	IMMINENT BIRTH
RESOURCES	BLS RESPONSE
C-SPINE	NO SIGNS OF TRAUMA

PATHOPHYSIOLOGY

Overview:

The management of labor and delivery outside of the hospital can be a stressful situation. It's important for providers to be prepared for imminent delivery and appropriately manage any complications that may occur. Assessing whether any pain is present, is there any vaginal bleeding and if contractions are occurring how strong and how far apart are they? History is very important: is this a repeat pregnant or birth for the patient, is this a multiple pregnancy, has the patient received any prenatal care? Recognizing when delivery is imminent and if transport is not recommended are critical. Crowning is a sign of imminent birth. The mother should be placed on her back with her knees widely separated the buttocks can be elevated with pillows. Providers should assist with head and shoulder delivery to prevent an explosive delivery. Coaching the mother to take slow deep breaths through her mouth will help to overcome the strong urge to push. Postpartum bleeding can sometimes be controlled by external uterine massage encouraging the uterus to clamp down. After placental delivery the mother should be encouraged to breast-feed. Transport should occur immediately. Essentials of newborn care include assessment, drying and heat conservation, proper positioning and physical stimulation to promote breathing.

Management of Breech Delivery:

Support the buttocks or extremities until the back appears. Grasp the baby's ILIAC WINGS and apply gentle downward traction. DO NOT pull on the legs or back, as this may cause spine dislocation or adrenal hemorrhage. Gently swing the infant's body in the direction of least resistance. By swinging anteriorly and posteriorly, both shoulders should deliver posteriorly. Splint the humerus bones with your two fingers; apply gentle traction with your fingers. Gentle downward compression of the uterus will assist in head delivery. Swing the legs upward until the body is in a vertical position. This will permit delivery of the head.

T3 SIMULATION SYSTEM

Normal Delivery-Performance

Performance Checklist | Role: | Start Time: | End Time:

Expected Actions	Time	2	1	0	N/A
1. Scene Size-up*					
2. Primary Survey: CC, LOC					
3. Primary Survey: ABCs					
4. SA: Pelvic Exam*					
5. Differential DX: Imminent*					
6. Transport: On scene del.*					
7. SA: Vitals					
8. Past Medical History					
9. Prepare Birth Field*					
10. Assist with Birth*					
12. Intervention: Warm & Dry*					
13. Assess Newborn : ABC					
14. APGAR 1 and 5 min.					
15. Transport: Non-emergent					
16. Reassessment					
17. Assess PPH					
18. Deliver Placenta					
19. Report					
TEAMWORK/LEADERSHIP					
1. Coordination					
2. Flexibility					
3. Communication					
4. Affect: Rapport & Support					
5. Overall					

*actions are mandatory

SELF EVALUATION: ☐ **Successful** ☐ **Unsuccessful** | **SCORE:** /48

NOTES:

Potentially Harmful/Dangerous Actions (omission, commission, sequencing):

C DEBRIEFING

10. Debriefing Questions:

1. How did you feel throughout the simulation experience?
2. What were your primary diagnoses in this scenario?
3. Did you feel you had the knowledge and skills to care for this patient? Why/ why not?
4. What were your priority assessments and interventions?
5. What outcomes did you measure?
6. What did you do well?
7. What was missed? What would you have done differently?

11. Critical Thinking

1. How do you know if birth is imminent? Active crowning, time between contractions, length of contractions, strength of contractions will all indicate birth is imminent.

2. Should this baby be delivered on scene or in the ambulance? It is preferable to deliver baby on scene but be prepared for rapid transport if complications arise.

Abnormal Delivery

Performance Checklist Role: Start Time: End Time:

Expected Actions	Time	2	1	0	N/A
1. Scene Size-up*					
2. Primary Survey: CC, LOC					
3. Primary Survey: ABCs					
4. SA: Pelvic Exam*					
5. Differential DX: Breech *					
6. Rapid Transport*					
7. SA: Vitals					
8. Past Medical History					
9. Prepare Birth Field*					
10. Assist with Birth*					
12. Intervention: Warm & Dry*					
13. Assess Newborn : ABC					
14. APGAR 1 and 5 min.					
16. Reassessment					
17. Assess PPH					
18. Deliver Placenta					
19. Report					
TEAMWORK/LEADERSHIP					
1. Coordination					
2. Flexibility					
3. Communication					
4. Affect: Rapport & Support					
5. Overall					

(*) actions are mandatory

SELF EVALUATION: ☐ Successful ☐ Unsuccessful **SCORE:** /48

NOTES:

Potentially Harmful/Dangerous Actions (omission, commission, sequencing):

C DEBRIEFING

Debriefing Questions:

1. How did you feel throughout the simulation experience?
2. What were your primary diagnoses in this scenario?
3. Did you feel you had the knowledge and skills to care for this patient? Why/ why not?
4. What were your priority assessments and interventions?
5. What outcomes did you measure?
6. What did you do well?
7. What was missed? What would you have done differently?

Critical Thinking

1. Why is breech presentation a complication?

2. If the baby cannot be delivered by EMS what actions are required?

EMS PATIENT CARE REPORT (PCR) Scenario:

PATIENT INFORMATION

Name:	Allergies:
Age:	Medications:
Sex:	Past Medical History:
Weight: Kg (lb)	Chief Complaint:

VITAL SIGNS

Time:	BP:	Pulse:	Respiration:	Sao_2:
Time:	BP:	Pulse:	Respiration:	Sao_2:
Time:	BP:	Pulse:	Respiration:	Sao_2:

PHYSICAL / NEUROLOGICAL EXAM

LOC:	Skin:	AB/GI:
Oriented:	HEENT:	Pelvis:
GCS:	Neck:	GU:
Pupils:	Chest:	Posterior :
Sensory/Motor:	Respiratory:	Extremities:
Facial Droop:	Cardiovascular:	Psychiatric:
Speech:	EKG:	GLU:

CHIEF COMPLAINT

HISTORY OF PRESENT ILLNESS

NOTES

EMS PATIENT CARE REPORT (PCR) Scenario:

PATIENT INFORMATION

Name:	Allergies:
Age:	Medications:
Sex:	Past Medical History:
Weight: Kg (lb)	Chief Complaint:

VITAL SIGNS

Time:	BP:	Pulse:	Respiration:	Sao_2:
Time:	BP:	Pulse:	Respiration:	Sao_2:
Time:	BP:	Pulse:	Respiration:	Sao_2:

PHYSICAL / NEUROLOGICAL EXAM

LOC:	Skin:	AB/GI:
Oriented:	HEENT:	Pelvis:
GCS:	Neck:	GU:
Pupils:	Chest:	Posterior :
Sensory/Motor:	Respiratory:	Extremities:
Facial Droop:	Cardiovascular:	Psychiatric:
Speech:	EKG:	GLU:

CHIEF COMPLAINT

HISTORY OF PRESENT ILLNESS

NOTES

NEONATE

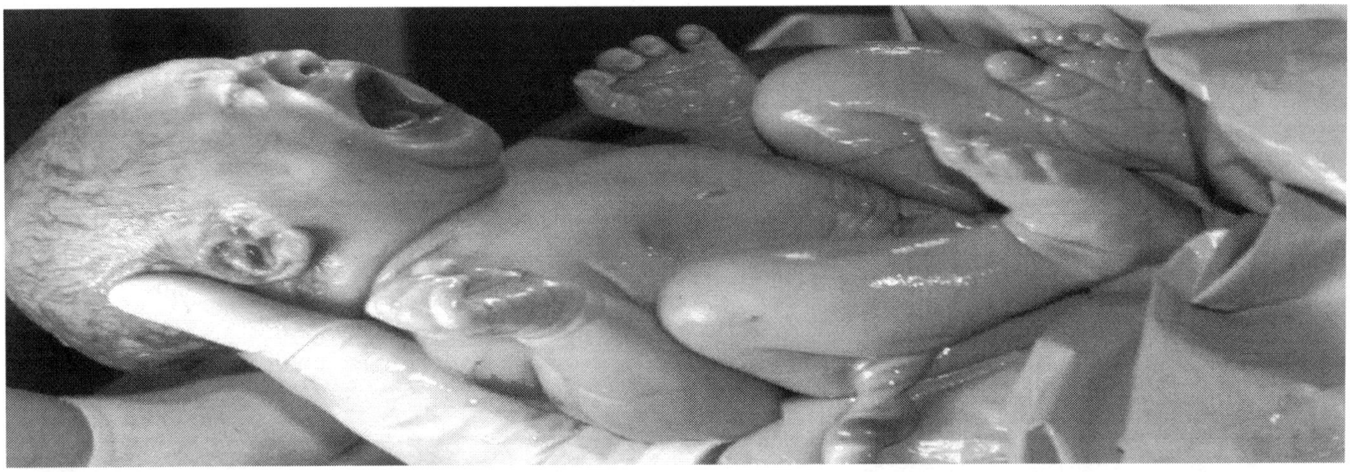

NEWBORN , NORMAL and UNRESPONSIVE

DISPATCH
Location: Suburban home
Type of situation: Newborn
Number of patients: 1
Hazards: No hazards

OBJECTIVES
1) Anticipates emergent delivery and prepares necessary equipment
2) Demonstrates an approach to fetal delivery & management of neonate
3) Appropriately manages the neonate using the NRP guidelines for O2 use, PPV, intubation, chest compressions and medications

SCENE SIZE-UP	
OVERALL SAFETY	SCENE IS SAFE
MOI / NOI	NEWBORN
RESOURCES	ALS RESPONSE
C-SPINE	NO SIGNS OF TRAUMA

PATHOPHYSIOLOGY

Overview:

Neonatal Resuscitation is intervention after a baby is born to help it breathe and to help its heart beat.

Before a baby is born, the placenta provides oxygen and nutrition to the blood and removes carbon dioxide. After a baby is born, the lungs provide oxygen to the blood and remove carbon dioxide.
The transition from using the placenta to using the lungs for gas exchange begins when the umbilical cord is clamped or tied off, and the baby has its first breath. Many babies go through this transition without needing intervention. Some babies need help with establishing their air flow, breathing, or circulation.
Resuscitation is helping with Airway, Breathing, and Circulation and the NRP inverted triangle.

Approximately 10% of newly born infants require some assistance to begin breathing. Deliveries complicated by maternal bleeding (placenta previa or placental abruption) place the infant at risk for hypovolemia secondary to blood loss. Low birth weight infants are at high risk for hypothermia due to heat loss. Normalization of blood oxygen levels ($SaO2$ 85-95%) will not be achieved until approximately 10 minutes following birth. Both hypoxia and excess oxygen administration can result in harm to the infant. If prolonged oxygen use is required, titrate to maintain an oxygen saturation of 85-95%. Increase in heart rate is the most reliable indicator of effective resuscitative efforts.

Acrocyanosis, a blue discoloration of the distal extremities, is a common finding in the newly born infant transitioning to extrauterine life. This must be differentiated from central cyanosis.

Proper resuscitation requires essential equipment and knowledge of necessary protocols before delivery. Prior knowledge of the gestational age of the newborn is helpful in anticipating the need for resuscitation. Low birth weight and premature delivery predispose infants to the need for resuscitative efforts.

Neonatal Resuscitation - HR>100

Performance Checklist | **Role:** | **Start Time:** **End Time:**

Expected Actions	Time	2	1	0	N/A
1. Clamp and cut umbilical cord					
2. Primary Survey: ABC					
3. TI: Warm and dry baby*					
4. SA: Sp02					
5. TI: Blow-by 100% O_2					
6. TI: Airway Management					
7. SA: Auscultate					
8. Place baby with mother					
9. Reassess :APGAR 1 and 5					
10. Report					
* Critical Actions					
TEAMWORK/LEADERSHIP					
1. Coordination					
2. Flexibility					
3. Communication					
4. Affect: Rapport & Support					
5. Overall					

SELF EVALUATION: ☐ Successful ☐ Unsuccessful

SCORE: /30

NOTES:

C DEBRIEFING

Debriefing Questions:

1.How did feel throughout the simulation experience?
2.What were your primary diagnoses in this scenario?
3.Did you feel you had the knowledge and skills to care for this patient? Why/ why not?
4.What were your priority assessments and interventions?
5.What outcomes did you measure?
6.What did you do well?
7.What was missed? What would you have done differently?
8.Is there anything else you would like to discuss?

Critical Thinking

1. What is assessed with APGAR scale?

2. Where should the pulse ox probe be placed on a neonate?

3. Compare and contrast central cyanosis and acrocyanosis.

Neonatal Resuscitation HR < 60

Performance Checklist Role: **Start Time:** **End Time:**

Expected Actions	Time	2	1	0	N/A
1. Clamp and cut umbilical cord					
2. Primary Survey: ABC					
3. TI: Warm and dry baby*					
4. SA: Sp02					
5. TI: Airway Management -suction					
6. TI: Airway adjunct					
7. TI: BVM 100% O2*					
8. TI: Chest compressions*					
9. TI: IV/IO *					
10. TI: Medications -Epi*					
11 . TI: Intubate *					
12. Rapid transport*					
13. Reassess					
14. Report					
TEAMWORK/LEADERSHIP					
1. Coordination					
2. Flexibility					
3. Communication					
4. Affect: Rapport & Support					
5. Overall					

SELF EVALUATION: ☐ Successful ☐ Unsuccessful

SCORE: /38

NOTES:

C DEBRIEFING

Debriefing Questions:

1.How did feel throughout the simulation experience?
2.What were your primary diagnoses in this scenario?
3.Did you feel you had the knowledge and skills to care for this patient? Why/ why not?
4.What were your priority assessments and interventions?
5.What outcomes did you measure?
6.What did you do well?
7.What was missed? What would you have done differently?
8.Is there anything else you would like to discuss?

Critical Thinking

1. What percentage of newborns will require resuscitation efforts?

2. Which intervention is most critical in a neonate?

EMS PATIENT CARE REPORT (PCR) Scenario:

PATIENT INFORMATION

Name:	Allergies:
Age:	Medications:
Sex:	Past Medical History:
Weight: Kg (lb)	Chief Complaint:

VITAL SIGNS

Time:	BP:	Pulse:	Respiration:	Sao_2:
Time:	BP:	Pulse:	Respiration:	Sao_2:
Time:	BP:	Pulse:	Respiration:	Sao_2:

PHYSICAL / NEUROLOGICAL EXAM

LOC:	Skin:	AB/GI:
Oriented:	HEENT:	Pelvis:
GCS:	Neck:	GU:
Pupils:	Chest:	Posterior :
Sensory/Motor:	Respiratory:	Extremities:
Facial Droop:	Cardiovascular:	Psychiatric:
Speech:	EKG:	GLU:

CHIEF COMPLAINT

HISTORY OF PRESENT ILLNESS

NOTES

EMS PATIENT CARE REPORT (PCR) Scenario:

PATIENT INFORMATION

Name: Age: Sex: Weight: Kg (lb)	Allergies: Medications: Past Medical History: Chief Complaint:

VITAL SIGNS

Time:	BP:	Pulse:	Respiration:	Sao_2:
Time:	BP:	Pulse:	Respiration:	Sao_2:
Time:	BP:	Pulse:	Respiration:	Sao_2:

PHYSICAL / NEUROLOGICAL EXAM

LOC:	Skin:	AB/GI:
Oriented:	HEENT:	Pelvis:
GCS:	Neck:	GU:
Pupils:	Chest:	Posterior :
Sensory/Motor:	Respiratory:	Extremities:
Facial Droop:	Cardiovascular:	Psychiatric:
Speech:	EKG:	GLU:

CHIEF COMPLAINT

HISTORY OF PRESENT ILLNESS

NOTES

PEDIATRIC ALLERGY / ANAPHYLAXIS

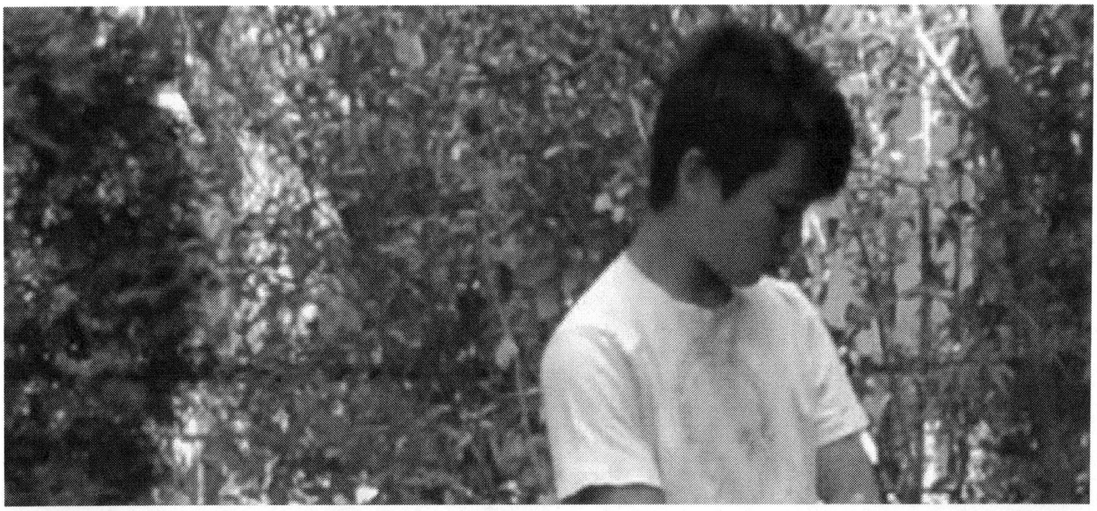

16 Y/O MALE, SHORTNESS OF BREATH AFTER BEE STING

DISPATCH
Location: Suburban backward
Type of situation: SOB after bee sting
Number of patients: 1
Hazards: No hazards

OBJECTIVES

1. Understand the pathophysiology of anaphylactic shock in pediatric patient.
2. Quickly assess and recognize anaphylaxis in pediatric patient.
3. Prioritize treatment for anaphylactic shock.
4. Appropriately manage patient's airway.
5. Exhibit teamwork and communication to evaluate and treat severe respiratory distress in children.

SCENE SIZE-UP	
OVERALL SAFETY	SCENE IS SAFE
MOI / NOI	SOB, BEE STING
RESOURCES	BLS RESPONSE
C-SPINE	NO SIGNS OF TRAUMA

PATHOPHYSIOLOGY

Overview:

Anaphylaxis is an acute, potentially life-threatening syndrome, with multisystem manifestations resulting from the rapid release of inflammatory agents. In children, foods can be a very significant trigger for anaphylaxis. Milk, eggs, wheat, and soy as a group are the most common food allergens; however, peanuts and fish are among the most potent. Environmental allergens and medications are also significant triggers.
The immune response ignites a cascade that results in the release and production of several inflammatory and vasoactive substances. In anaphylaxis, these substances most commonly involve the skin, respiratory, cardiovascular, and gastrointestinal systems. As a result, rashes, angioedema, bronchospasm, laryngospasm, increased vascular permeability and decreased vascular tone, and bloody diarrhea can develop. In addition respiratory compromise (eg, bronchospasm, stridor, shortness of breath) and/or reduced blood pressure or associated symptoms of end-organ dysfunction (eg, syncope, incontinence) can also be present.
The early use of epinephrine is the most important step in managing anaphylaxis. Prehospital care should be directed at stabilization of the airway, breathing, and circulation (the "ABCs"). In addition, intravenous (IV) access should be obtained; intraosseous (IO) access should be considered when IV access cannot be-

quickly obtained in unstable patients.

Pediatric Anaphylaxis: Performance

Performance Checklist **Role:** | **Start Time:** **End Time:**

Expected Actions	Time	2	1	0	N/A
1. Scene size-up: Address Safety*					
2. PS- CC, LOC, HPI*					
3. PS- ABC*					
4. TI: 100% 02 NRB*					
5. SA: Past Medical History*					
6. Secondary Asses.: Vital Signs					
7. Differential Diagnosis:Anaphylaxis*					
8. Ti- Epi 1:1000 IM*					
9. Transport: Non-emergent					
10. Reass: ABC, Vitals, Pt Monitor					
11. TI:Nebulizer treatment;IV Access*					
12. Recognize Deterioration*					
13. TI: BVM*					
14. Communication:Medical Control					
16. TI: EPI 1:1000 IM; IV Fluids*					
17. TI: Meds Benadryl & Solumedrol					
18. Reassessment					
TEAMWORK/LEADERSHIP					
1. Coordination					
2. Flexibility					
3. Communication					
4. Affect: Rapport & Support*					
5. Overall					

*Actions are mandatory

SELF EVALUATION: ☐ **Successful** ☐ **Unsuccessful** | **SCORE: /46**

NOTES:

Potentially Harmful/ Dangerous Actions (omission, commission, sequencing):

C DEBRIEFING

10. Debriefing Questions:

1. How did feel throughout the simulation experience?
2. What were your primary diagnoses in this scenario?
3. Did you feel you had the knowledge and skills to care for this patient? Why/ why not?
4. What were your priority assessments and interventions?
5. What outcomes did you measure?
6. What did you do well?
7. What was missed? What would you have done differently?
8. Is there anything else you would like to discuss?
9. Ask these questions during the video debriefing.

11. Critical Thinking

1. How serious is this patient, why?
2. What can cause an anaphylactic patient to become hypotensive?

Pediatric Anaphylaxis: Performance

Performance Checklist Role: | **Start Time:** **End Time:**

Expected Actions	Time	2	1	0	N/A
1. Scene size-up: Address Safety*					
2. PS- CC, LOC, HPI*					
3. PS- ABC*					
4. TI: 100% 02 NRB*					
5. Past Medical History*					
6. Secondary Asses.: Vital Signs					
7. Differential Diagnosis:*					
8. TI:*					
9. Transport:					
10. Reass: ABC, Vitals, Pt Monitor					
11. TI:*					
12. Recognize Deterioration*					
13. TI: *					
14. Communication:Medical Control					
16. TI:*					
17. TI:					
18. Reassessment					
19. Report					
TEAMWORK/LEADERSHIP					
1. Coordination					
2. Flexibility					
3. Communication					
4. Affect: Rapport & Support*					
5. Overall					

RED Actions are mandatory*

SELF EVALUATION: ☐ **Successful** ☐ **Unsuccessful** | **SCORE:** /48

NOTES:

Potentially Harmful/ Dangerous Actions (omission, commission, sequencing):

C DEBRIEFING

10. Debriefing Questions:

1. How did feel throughout the simulation experience?

2. What were your primary diagnoses in this scenario?

3. Did you feel you had the knowledge and skills to care for this patient? Why/ why not?

4. What were your priority assessments and interventions?

5. What outcomes did you measure?

6. What did you do well?

7. What was missed? What would you have done differently?

8. Is there anything else you would like to discuss?

9. Ask these questions during the video debriefing.

11. Critical Thinking

1. How serious is the patient?

2. Distinguish between allergic and anaphylactic reactions in terms of pathophysiology and care?

EMS PATIENT CARE REPORT (PCR) Scenario:

PATIENT INFORMATION

Name: Age: Sex: Weight: Kg (lb)	Allergies: Medications: Past Medical History: Chief Complaint:

VITAL SIGNS

Time:	BP:	Pulse:	Respiration:	Sao_2:
Time:	BP:	Pulse:	Respiration:	Sao_2:
Time:	BP:	Pulse:	Respiration:	Sao_2:

PHYSICAL / NEUROLOGICAL EXAM

LOC:	Skin:	AB/GI:
Oriented:	HEENT:	Pelvis:
GCS:	Neck:	GU:
Pupils:	Chest:	Posterior :
Sensory/Motor:	Respiratory:	Extremities:
Facial Droop:	Cardiovascular:	Psychiatric:
Speech:	EKG:	GLU:

CHIEF COMPLAINT

HISTORY OF PRESENT ILLNESS

NOTES

EMS PATIENT CARE REPORT (PCR) Scenario:

PATIENT INFORMATION

Name: Age: Sex: Weight: Kg (lb)	Allergies: Medications: Past Medical History: Chief Complaint:

VITAL SIGNS

Time:	BP:	Pulse:	Respiration:	Sao_2:
Time:	BP:	Pulse:	Respiration:	Sao_2:
Time:	BP:	Pulse:	Respiration:	Sao_2:

PHYSICAL / NEUROLOGICAL EXAM

LOC:	Skin:	AB/GI:
Oriented:	HEENT:	Pelvis:
GCS:	Neck:	GU:
Pupils:	Chest:	Posterior :
Sensory/Motor:	Respiratory:	Extremities:
Facial Droop:	Cardiovascular:	Psychiatric:
Speech:	EKG:	GLU:

CHIEF COMPLAINT

HISTORY OF PRESENT ILLNESS

NOTES

PEDIATRIC RESPIRATORY

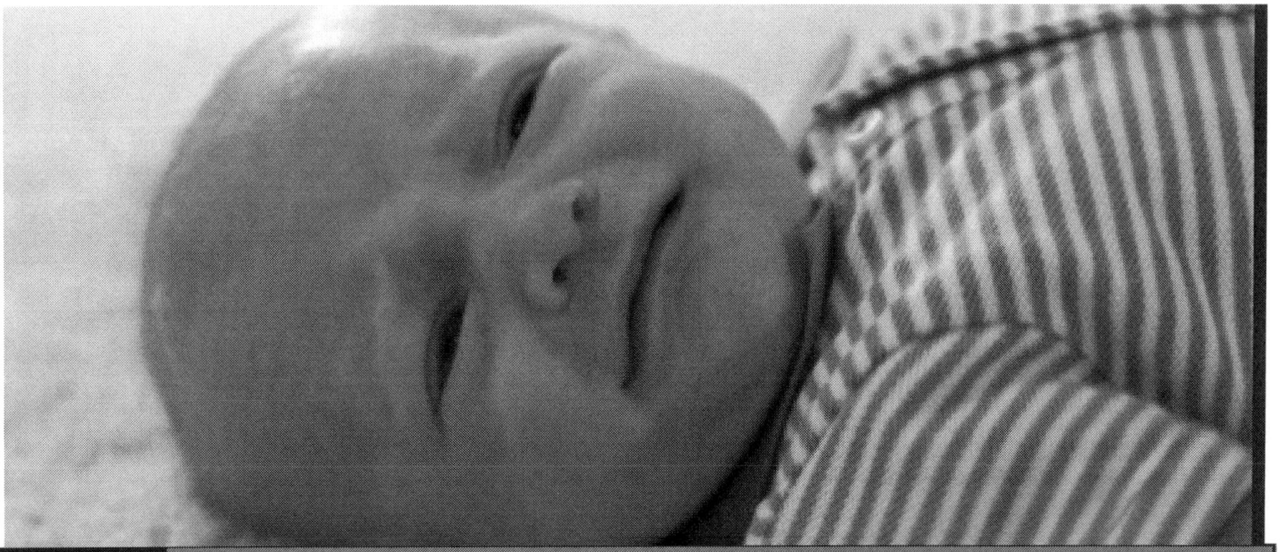

20 M/O FEMALE, DIFFICULTY BREATHING

DISPATCH
Location: Suburban home
Type of situation: Wheeze and SOB
Number of patients: 1
Hazards: No hazards

OBJECTIVES

a. Understand the pathophysiology of asthma and respiratory distress in children
b. Recognize asthma in children.
c. Recognition impending respiratory failure in children.
d. Prioritization of treatment.
e. How to correctly BVM a child with respiratory failure.
f. Exhibit teamwork and communication to evaluate and treat severe respiratory distress in children.

SCENE SIZE-UP	
OVERALL SAFETY	SCENE IS SAFE
MOI / NOI	WHEEZE ANS SOB
RESOURCES	ALS RESPONSE
C-SPINE	NO SIGNS OF TRAUMA

PATHOPHYSIOLOGY

Overview:

Respiratory distress in children and infants is serious and can be fatal. The responder must be able to rapidly assess the level of distress as well as the level of fatigue of the patient.

Respiratory distress can be caused by the interruption of air going into the lungs (upper airway obstruction), difficulty in getting exhaled air out of the lungs (lower airway obstruction), or damage to the lung tissue itself (pneumonia).
Lower airway obstruction is most commonly asthma. Asthma is acute inflammation of the bronchioles and smaller bronchi. Asthma is episodic and is usually triggered by an event such as an upper respiratory infection, allergen, cold weather, or secondhand smoke. The resulting inflammation results in bronchoconstriction, mucus production, and airway swelling. Air-trapping occurs as the ability to exhale is diminished due to the narrowed airways. Symptoms are wheezing, expiratory initially, then inspiratory. Regardless of the cause, it is critical to identify the patient that has respiratory fatigue and impending respiratory failure.
Signs and symptoms of impending respiratory failure are:Tachycardia (early sign), tachypnea, nasal flaring, retractions of respiratory muscles, agitation, anxiety, irritability, skin pallor, silent chest (late), cyanosis (late), decreased LOC (late) Bradycardia (late), Bradypnea (late), thoracic-abdominal movement (seesawing) (very late).

Aggressive and immediate treatment must occur to prevent respiratory and circulatory failure. Oxygen in high concentrations, keep SaO2 above 94%, Administer albuterol MDI or nebulizer, Administer Epinephrine via Epi-Pen or IM injection. Administer atrovent via nebulizer,and Solu-Medrol IV. Consider BVM or Intubation

Pediatric Asthma: Performance

Performance Checklist Role:

Start Time: **End Time:**

Expected Actions	Time	2	1	0	N/A
1. Scene SU: Address Safety *					
2. PS - CC, LOC, HPI					
3. PS: ABC					
4. TI: 100% 02 NB					
5. Past Medical History					
6. SA: Vital Signs					
7.. DD: Asthma Exacerbation *					
8. TI: Nebulizer Treatment *					
9. Affect: Rapport					
10. Transport: Non-Emergent					
11. Reass: ABC, Vitals, Monitor					
12. Recognize Deterioration *					
13. TI: BVM *					
14. TI: EPI 1:1000 *					
15. Communication: Med Cont					
16. TI: IV Access/ Fluids					
17. TI: MgSO4 & Solumedrol					
18. TI Intubation *					
TEAMWORK/LEADERSHIP					
1. Coordination					
2. Flexibility					
3. Communication					
4. Affect: Rapport & Support *					
5. Overall					

(*) actions are mandatory

SELF EVALUATION: ☐ **Successful** ☐ **Unsuccessful**

SCORE: /46

NOTES:

Potentially Harmful/ Dangerous Actions (omission, commission, sequencing):

C DEBRIEFING

10. Debriefing Questions:

1. How did feel throughout the simulation experience?
2. What were your primary diagnoses in this scenario?
3. Did you feel you had the knowledge and skills to care for this patient? Why/ why not?
4. What were your priority assessments and interventions?
5. What outcomes did you measure?
6. What did you do well?
7. What was missed? What would you have done differently?
8. Is there anything else you would like to discuss?
9. Ask these questions during the video debriefing.

11. Critical Thinking

1. How serious is this patient, why?-

2. What other treatment is available?

3. When do you need to take over the respiratory efforts?

T3 SIMULATION SYSTEM

Pediatric Respiratory Failure

Performance Checklist Role: | Start Time: End Time:

Expected Actions	Time	2	1	0	N/A
1. Scene SU: Address Safety *					
2. PS - CC, LOC, HPI					
3. PS: ABC					
4. TI: 100% 02 NB					
5. Past Medical History					
6. SA: Vital Signs/Monitor					
7.. DD: Asthma Exacerbation *					
8. TI: Nebulizer Treatment *					
9. Affect: Rapport					
10. Transport: Emergent					
11. Reass: ABC, Vitals, Monitor					
12. Recognize Deterioration *					
13. TI: BVM *					
14. TI: EPI 1:1000 *					
15. Communication: Med Cont					
16. Recognize Deterioration *					
17. TI: Intubate*					
18. Report					
TEAMWORK/LEADERSHIP					
1. Coordination					
2. Flexibility					
3. Communication					
4. Affect: Rapport & Support *					
5. Overall					

(*) actions are mandatory

SELF EVALUATION: ☐ Successful ☐ Unsuccessful | **SCORE:** /46

NOTES:

Potentially Harmful/ Dangerous Actions (omission, commission, sequencing):

C DEBRIEFING

Debriefing Questions:

1. How did feel throughout the simulation experience?
2. What were your primary diagnoses in this scenario?
3. Did you feel you had the knowledge and skills to care for this patient? Why/ why not?
4. What were your priority assessments and interventions?
5. What outcomes did you measure?
6. What did you do well?
7. What was missed? What would you have done differently?
8. Is there anything else you would like to discuss?
9. Ask these questions during the video debriefing.

Critical Thinking

1. Do the following clinical signs represent respiratory distress or respiratory failure? Marked tachypnea, bradycardia, cyanosis, and poor air movement.

2. When there are signs of respiratory distress or respiratory failure, the first priority is ?

EMS PATIENT CARE REPORT (PCR) Scenario:

PATIENT INFORMATION

Name:	Allergies:
Age:	Medications:
Sex:	Past Medical History:
Weight: Kg (lb)	Chief Complaint:

VITAL SIGNS

Time:	BP:	Pulse:	Respiration:	Sao_2:
Time:	BP:	Pulse:	Respiration:	Sao_2:
Time:	BP:	Pulse:	Respiration:	Sao_2:

PHYSICAL / NEUROLOGICAL EXAM

LOC:	Skin:	AB/GI:
Oriented:	HEENT:	Pelvis:
GCS:	Neck:	GU:
Pupils:	Chest:	Posterior :
Sensory/Motor:	Respiratory:	Extremities:
Facial Droop:	Cardiovascular:	Psychiatric:
Speech:	EKG:	GLU:

CHIEF COMPLAINT

HISTORY OF PRESENT ILLNESS

NOTES

EMS PATIENT CARE REPORT (PCR) Scenario:

PATIENT INFORMATION

Name:	Allergies:
Age:	Medications:
Sex:	Past Medical History:
Weight: Kg (lb)	Chief Complaint:

VITAL SIGNS

Time:	BP:	Pulse:	Respiration:	Sao_2:
Time:	BP:	Pulse:	Respiration:	Sao_2:
Time:	BP:	Pulse:	Respiration:	Sao_2:

PHYSICAL / NEUROLOGICAL EXAM

LOC:	Skin:	AB/GI:
Oriented:	HEENT:	Pelvis:
GCS:	Neck:	GU:
Pupils:	Chest:	Posterior :
Sensory/Motor:	Respiratory:	Extremities:
Facial Droop:	Cardiovascular:	Psychiatric:
Speech:	EKG:	GLU:

CHIEF COMPLAINT

HISTORY OF PRESENT ILLNESS

NOTES

PEDIATRIC BLUNT TRAUMA

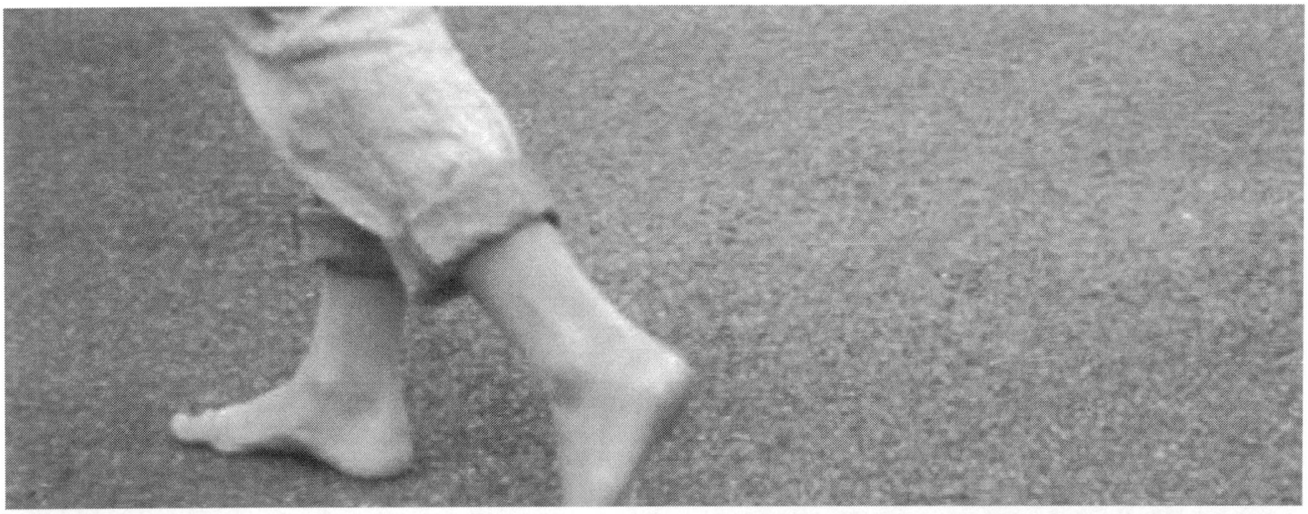

2 Y/O FEMALE UNRESPONSIVE

DISPATCH
Location: Suburban home
Type of situation: MVA
Time of Day: 01:00 pm
Number of patients: 1
Hazards: Scene is safe

OBJECTIVES

a. Assessment of the critically injured patient
b. Understand pathophysiology of tension pneumothorax
c. Prioritize interventions using critical thinking
d. Recognize and treat tension pneumothorax
e. Recognition and treatment of hypovolemic shock
f. Use of long spine board for immobilization/evacuation
g. Demonstrate effective teamwork

SCENE SIZE-UP	
OVERALL SAFETY	SCENE IS SAFE
MOI / NOI	MVA
RESOURCES	ALS RESPONSE
C-SPINE	SIGNS OF TRAUMA

PATHOPHYSIOLOGY

Overview:

A traumatic pneumothorax may result from both blunt trauma and penetrating injuries to the chest wall. The most common mechanism is a cut to the pleura by a fractured rib. Tension pneumothorax occurs because the opening that allows air to enter the pleural space functions like a valve, and with every breath more air enters and cannot escape. Severe hypoxia follows, with a resultant drop in blood pressure and level of consciousness.

Signs and symptoms of a Tension Pneumothorax is severe respiratory distress, low blood pressure, JVD, absent lung sounds on the affected side, muffled heart sounds, subcutaneous emphysema, and a late sign of tracheal deviation. A tension pneumo is treated with needle chest decompression at either the 2nd intercostals space over the top of the third rib midclavicular, or the 5th intercostals space mid axillary. Due to the potential underlying injuries with no exit wound spinal precautions are necessary.

Pediatric Tension Pneumothorax-

Performance Checklist Role:

Start Time: End Time:

Expected Actions	Time	2	1	0	N/A
1. Scene Size-up: Safety					
2. Primary Survey: CC, LOC, HPI					
3. Primary Survey: ABCs					
4. Spinal immobilization					
5. Primary Assessment					
6. Administer O_2 by NRB at 15 lpm*					
7. Perform NCD*					
8. Start IV					
9. Appropriate transport decision					
10. Reassessment					
11. Report					
* Critical Actions					
TEAMWORK/LEADERSHIP					
1. Coordination					
2. Flexibility					
3. Communication					
4. Affect: Rapport & Support					
5. Overall					

SELF EVALUATION: ☐ Successful ☐ Unsuccessful

SCORE: /32

NOTES:

C DEBRIEFING

Debriefing Questions:

1. What happened?
2. How did you feel throughout the simulation experience?
3. What were your priority assessments and interventions?
4. What did you do well? What was missed? What would you have done differently?
5. What was going to save this patient's life?
6. Anything else you would like to discuss?

Critical Thinking

1. What is the one physiologic aspect of a child's thorax that makes an injury pattern different than an adult with similar mechanism of injury?

2. Discuss the need for intubation with this patient.

Pediatric Blunt Trauma

Performance Checklist **Role:** **Start Time:** **End Time:**

Expected Actions	Time	2	1	0	N/A
1. Scene Size-up: Safety					
2. Primary Survey: CC, LOC, HPI					
3. Primary Survey: ABCs					
4. Spinal immobilization					
5. Primary Assessment					
6. Administer O_2 by NRB at 15 lpm					
7. TI:					
8. TI: Start IV					
9. Appropriate transport decision					
10. Reassessment					
11. TI:					
12. Report					
TEAMWORK/LEADERSHIP					
1. Coordination					
2. Flexibility					
3. Communication					
4. Affect: Rapport & Support					
5. Overall					

SELF EVALUATION: ☐ Successful ☐ Unsuccessful

SCORE: /34

NOTES:

C DEBRIEFING

Debriefing Questions:

1. What happened?
2. How did you feel throughout the simulation experience?
3. What were your priority assessments and interventions?
4. What did you do well? What was missed? What would you have done differently?
5. What was going to save this patient's life?
6. Anything else you would like to discuss?

Critical Thinking

1. What is the most common cause of death in children under 14 years of age?

2. Discuss fluid administration in pediatric patients.

EMS PATIENT CARE REPORT (PCR) Scenario:

PATIENT INFORMATION

Name:	Allergies:
Age:	Medications:
Sex:	Past Medical History:
Weight: Kg (lb)	Chief Complaint:

VITAL SIGNS

Time:	BP:	Pulse:	Respiration:	Sao_2:
Time:	BP:	Pulse:	Respiration:	Sao_2:
Time:	BP:	Pulse:	Respiration:	Sao_2:

PHYSICAL / NEUROLOGICAL EXAM

LOC:	Skin:	AB/GI:
Oriented:	HEENT:	Pelvis:
GCS:	Neck:	GU:
Pupils:	Chest:	Posterior :
Sensory/Motor:	Respiratory:	Extremities:
Facial Droop:	Cardiovascular:	Psychiatric:
Speech:	EKG:	GLU:

CHIEF COMPLAINT

HISTORY OF PRESENT ILLNESS

NOTES

EMS PATIENT CARE REPORT (PCR) Scenario:

PATIENT INFORMATION

Name:	Allergies:
Age:	Medications:
Sex:	Past Medical History:
Weight: Kg (lb)	Chief Complaint:

VITAL SIGNS

Time:	BP:	Pulse:	Respiration:	Sao_2:
Time:	BP:	Pulse:	Respiration:	Sao_2:
Time:	BP:	Pulse:	Respiration:	Sao_2:

PHYSICAL / NEUROLOGICAL EXAM

LOC:	Skin:	AB/GI:
Oriented:	HEENT:	Pelvis:
GCS:	Neck:	GU:
Pupils:	Chest:	Posterior :
Sensory/Motor:	Respiratory:	Extremities:
Facial Droop:	Cardiovascular:	Psychiatric:
Speech:	EKG:	GLU:

CHIEF COMPLAINT

HISTORY OF PRESENT ILLNESS

NOTES

T3 SIMULATION SYSTEM

Scenario Checklist

Performance Checklist **Role:** **Start Time:** **End Time:**

Expected Actions	Time	2	1	0	N/A
1. Scene size-up *					
2. PS: ABCs					
3. TI :					
4. SA: Vitals					
5. SA: PMH					
6. Differential DX: *					
7. TI:					
8. Reassessment incl monitor					
9. Transport					
10. Reassessment*					
11. TI:*					
12. TI:*					
13. Reassessment					
14. TI*:					
15. Report					
TEAMWORK/LEADERSHIP					
1. Coordination of Treatment					
2. Communication					
3. Situational Awareness					
4. Affect					
5. Overall					

SELF EVALUATION: ☐ **Successful** ☐ **Unsuccessful**

SCORE: /40

NOTES: including Critical Items

Scenario Checklist

Performance Checklist | Role: | Start Time: End Time:

Expected Actions	Time	2	1	0	N/A
1. Scene size-up *					
2. PS: ABCs					
3. TI :					
4. SA: Vitals					
5. SA: PMH					
6. Differential DX: *					
7. TI:					
8. Reassessment incl monitor					
9. Transport					
10. Reassessment*					
11. TI:*					
12. TI:*					
13. Reassessment					
14. TI*:					
15. Report					
TEAMWORK/LEADERSHIP					
1. Coordination of Treatment					
2. Communication					
3. Situational Awareness					
4. Affect					
5. Overall					

SELF EVALUATION: ☐ Successful ☐ Unsuccessful

SCORE: /40

NOTES: including Critical Items

SIMULATION SYSTEM

Scenario Checklist

Performance Checklist Role: | **Start Time:** **End Time:**

Expected Actions	Time	2	1	0	N/A
1. Scene size-up *					
2. PS: ABCs					
3. TI :					
4. SA: Vitals					
5. SA: PMH					
6. Differential DX: *					
7. TI:					
8. Reassessment incl monitor					
9. Transport					
10. Reassessment*					
11. TI:*					
12. TI:*					
13. Reassessment					
14. TI*:					
15. Report					

TEAMWORK/LEADERSHIP					
1. Coordination of Treatment					
2. Communication					
3. Situational Awareness					
4. Affect					
5. Overall					

SELF EVALUATION: ☐ **Successful** ☐ **Unsuccessful**

SCORE: /40

NOTES: including Critical Items

Scenario Checklist

T3 SIMULATION SYSTEM

Performance Checklist	Role:	Start Time:	End Time:

Expected Actions	Time	2	1	0	N/A
1. Scene size-up *					
2. PS: ABCs					
3. TI :					
4. SA: Vitals					
5. SA: PMH					
6. Differential DX: *					
7. TI:					
8. Reassessment incl monitor					
9. Transport					
10. Reassessment*					
11. TI:*					
12. TI:*					
13. Reassessment					
14. TI*:					
15. Report					
TEAMWORK/LEADERSHIP					
1. Coordination of Treatment					
2. Communication					
3. Situational Awareness					
4. Affect					
5. Overall					

SELF EVALUATION: ☐ **Successful** ☐ **Unsuccessful**

SCORE: /40

NOTES: including Critical Items

Scenario Checklist

T3 SIMULATION SYSTEM

Performance Checklist **Role:** **Start Time:** **End Time:**

Expected Actions	Time	2	1	0	N/A
1. Scene size-up *					
2. PS: ABCs					
3. TI :					
4. SA: Vitals					
5. SA: PMH					
6. Differential DX: *					
7. TI:					
8. Reassessment incl monitor					
9. Transport					
10. Reassessment*					
11. TI:*					
12. TI:*					
13. Reassessment					
14. TI*:					
15. Report					
TEAMWORK/LEADERSHIP					
1. Coordination of Treatment					
2. Communication					
3. Situational Awareness					
4. Affect					
5. Overall					

SELF EVALUATION: ☐ **Successful** ☐ **Unsuccessful**

SCORE: /40

NOTES: including Critical Items

Scenario Checklist

T3 Simulation System

Performance Checklist | Role: | Start Time: | End Time:

Expected Actions	Time	2	1	0	N/A
1. Scene size-up *					
2. PS: ABCs					
3. TI :					
4. SA: Vitals					
5. SA: PMH					
6. Differential DX: *					
7. TI:					
8. Reassessment incl monitor					
9. Transport					
10. Reassessment*					
11. TI:*					
12. TI:*					
13. Reassessment					
14. TI*:					
15. Report					
TEAMWORK/LEADERSHIP					
1. Coordination of Treatment					
2. Communication					
3. Situational Awareness					
4. Affect					
5. Overall					

SELF EVALUATION: ☐ Successful ☐ Unsuccessful

SCORE: /40

NOTES: including Critical Items

T3 SIMULATION SYSTEM

Scenario Checklist

Performance Checklist | **Role:** | **Start Time:** **End Time:**

Expected Actions	Time	2	1	0	N/A
1. Scene size-up *					
2. PS: ABCs					
3. TI :					
4. SA: Vitals					
5. SA: PMH					
6. Differential DX: *					
7. TI:					
8. Reassessment incl monitor					
9. Transport					
10. Reassessment*					
11. TI:*					
12. TI:*					
13. Reassessment					
14. TI*:					
15. Report					
TEAMWORK/LEADERSHIP					
1. Coordination of Treatment					
2. Communication					
3. Situational Awareness					
4. Affect					
5. Overall					

SELF EVALUATION: ☐ Successful ☐ Unsuccessful

SCORE: /40

NOTES: including Critical Items

Scenario Checklist

T3 SIMULATION SYSTEM

Performance Checklist

Start Time: End Time:

Expected Actions	Time	2	1	0	N/A
1. Scene size-up *					
2. PS: ABCs					
3. TI :					
4. SA: Vitals					
5. SA: PMH					
6. Differential DX: *					
7. TI:					
8. Reassessment incl monitor					
9. Transport					
10. Reassessment*					
11. TI:*					
12. TI:*					
13. Reassessment					
14. TI*:					
15. Report					
TEAMWORK/LEADERSHIP					
1. Coordination of Treatment					
2. Communication					
3. Situational Awareness					
4. Affect					
5. Overall					

SELF EVALUATION: ☐ Successful ☐ Unsuccessful

SCORE: /40

NOTES: including Critical Items

T3 SIMULATION SYSTEM

Scenario Checklist

Performance Checklist

Start Time: **End Time:**

Expected Actions	Time	2	1	0	N/A
1. Scene size-up *					
2. PS: ABCs					
3. TI :					
4. SA: Vitals					
5. SA: PMH					
6. Differential DX: *					
7. TI:					
8. Reassessment incl monitor					
9. Transport					
10. Reassessment*					
11. TI:*					
12. TI:*					
13. Reassessment					
14. TI*:					
15. Report					
TEAMWORK/LEADERSHIP					
1. Coordination of Treatment					
2. Communication					
3. Situational Awareness					
4. Affect					
5. Overall					

SELF EVALUATION: ☐ **Successful** ☐ **Unsuccessful**

SCORE: **/40**

NOTES: including Critical Items

PART 2

SCENARIO AND SKILLS TRACKING

T3 Scenario Skills Map

SCENARIO	AIRWAY	IV / MEDS	CARDIAC	TRAUMA/MISC
ADULT Cardiac	BVM - Intubation	IV	12 Lead, Defib Cardioversion	
ADULT Diabetic		IV, Glucometer	EKG	
ADULT Overdose	BVM - Intubation	IV	12 Lead	
ADULT Psychiatric		IV/IM	EKG	Restraints
ADULT Seizure	BVM - Intubation	IV	EKG	
ADULT Trauma - Soft Tissue Burn	BVM - Intubation	IV	12 Lead, Pacing	
ADULT Trauma - Blunt Head	BVM - Intubation	IV		Immobilization
ADULT Trauma - Heat Emergency	BVM - Intubation	IV	EKG, CPR	
ADULT Trauma- Multi-System	BVM - Intubation	IV	12 Lead	Pelvic Binder Tourniquet
ADULT Trauma - Partial Amputation	BVM	IV	12 Lead	Tourniquet
ADULT Trauma- Penetrating GSW	BVM - Intubation	IV	EKG	NCD, Surgical Airway
GERIATRIC Abdominal Pain	BVM - Intubation	IV	12 Lead, Defib Pacing , CPR	
GERIATRIC Cardiac	BVM - Intubation	IV	12 Lead, Defib Pacing , CPR	
GERIATRIC Respiratory	BVM - Intubation CPAP	IV	12 Lead	
GERIATRIC Sepsis	BVM	IV	12 Lead	
GERIATRIC Stroke	BVM	IV	12 Lead	

T3 Scenario Skills Map

SCENARIO	AIRWAY	IV / MEDS	CARDIAC	TRAUMA
OB-GYN Delivery	BVM - Intubation	IV	12 Lead, Defib Cardioversion	
NEONATE Resuscitation	BVM - Intubation	IV/IO	CPR	
PEDIATRIC Allergy / Anaphylaxis	BVM - Intubation	IV/IO		
PEDIATRIC Respiratory	BVM - Intubation	IV/IO		
PEDIATRIC Trauma Blunt	BVM - Intubation	IV/IO	CPR	Needle Chest Decompression

Scenario Tracking Grid

Indicate Date / **P**ass or **F**ail

	ADULT-LEAD	MEMBER	GERI-LEAD	MEMBER	PEDS -LEAD	MEMBER
Respiratory Distress / Failure						
Chest Pain						
Cardiac Dysrthythmia/ Arrest						
Stroke						
Overdose / Poisoning						
Abdominal Pain						
Allergic Reaction						
Hypoglycemia / DKA/ HHNS						
Psychiatric						
Seizure						
Obstetric or Gynecologic						
Delivery w Neonatal Resuscitation						
Trauma (blunt, penetrating, burn, hemorrhage, enviro)						
Shock						
Sepsis						
Elective						

Scenario Tracking Grid

Indicate Date / **P**ass or **F**ail

	ADULT-LEAD	MEMBER	GERI-LEAD	MEMBER	PEDS -LEAD	MEMBER
Respiratory Distress / Failure						
Chest Pain						
Cardiac Dysrthythmia/ Arrest						
Stroke						
Overdose / Poisoning						
Abdominal Pain						
Allergic Reaction						
Hypoglycemia / DKA/ HHNS						
Psychiatric						
Seizure						
Obstetric or Gynecologic						
Delivery w Neonatal Resuscitation						
Trauma (blunt, penetrating, burn, hemorrhage, enviro)						
Shock						
Sepsis						
Elective						

T3 SIMULATION SYSTEM

Skills Tracking Grid

Individual Skills

Indicate date/ setting: **L**ab, **S**cenario, **P**atient, **C**linical

Attempt #	1	2	3	4	5	6	7	8	9	10
Patient History										
Physical Assessment - Adult										
Physical Assessment - Pediatric										
Orotracheal Intubation - Adult										
Orotracheal Intubation - Pediatric										
Nasotracheal Intubation - Adult										
Supraglottic Airway Device										
Needle Cricothyrotomy										
CPAP and PEEP										
Trauma Physical Assessment -Adult										
Trauma Endotracheal Intubation										
Pleural Decompression										
Intravenous Bolus										
Intravenous Piggyback Infusion										
IM and SubQ Medication Admin										
Intraosseous Infusion										
Synchronized Cardioversion										
12-Lead ECG Placement										
Defibrillation										
Transcutaneous Pacing										
Normal Delivery with Newborn Care										
Abnormal Delivery w Newborn Care										
Neonatal Resuscitation										

Skills Tracking Grid

Individual Skills

Indicate date/ setting: **L**ab, **S**cenario, **P**atient, **C**linical

Attempt #	1	2	3	4	5	6	7	8	9	10
Patient History										
Physical Assessment - Adult										
Physical Assessment - Pediatric										
Orotracheal Intubation - Adult										
Orotracheal Intubation - Pediatric										
Nasotracheal Intubation - Adult										
Supraglottic Airway Device										
Needle Cricothyrotomy										
CPAP and PEEP										
Trauma Physical Assessment -Adult										
Trauma Endotracheal Intubation										
Pleural Decompression										
Intravenous Bolus										
Intravenous Piggyback Infusion										
IM and SubQ Medication Admin										
Intraosseous Infusion										
Synchronized Cardioversion										
12-Lead ECG Placement										
Defibrillation										
Transcutaneous Pacing										
Normal Delivery with Newborn Care										
Abnormal Delivery w Newborn Care										
Neonatal Resuscitation										

Skills Tracking Grid

Individual Skills

Indicate date/ setting: **L**ab, **S**cenario, **P**atient, **C**linical

Attempt #	1	2	3	4	5	6	7	8	9	10
Medical with Cardiac Assessment										
Intravenous Therapy										

Skills Tracking Grid

Individual Skills

Indicate date/ setting: **L**ab, **S**cenario, **P**atient, **C**linical

Attempt #	1	2	3	4	5	6	7	8	9	10
Medical with Cardiac Assessment										
Intravenous Therapy										

Made in the USA
Monee, IL
05 November 2026

67385929R10116